LAUGHING IN THE DARK

*"A joyful heart is good medicine,
but a broken spirit dries up the bones."
Proverbs 17:22
(New American Standard Bible)*

Copyright © 2014 by Samuel L Thompson
All Rights Reserved

Cover photo by Kt Jane Photography

ISBN-13: 978-1503200012
ISBN-10: 1503200019

DEDICATION

I wish to dedicate this book to the memory of my mother, Nona Jane Thompson, who showed me how to laugh. As you read these pages, you will see just how much she has influenced my life.

Secondly, to my wife Ann, who has served as the inspiration and motivation for this book. She has taught me so much about what love and laughter really are.

Thirdly, to my brother Dale, whom I have laughed with, and at, as only brothers can. You will see in the pages of this book the close relationship Dale and I have shared.

Finally, I wish to dedicate this book to my Lord and Savior, Jesus Christ. It is my hope that it will point people to Him, for He is the only source of genuine laughter.

ACKNOWLEDGEMENTS

As any author knows, a book does not come about simply by sitting and typing. There are many people throughout its creation who contribute to its completion. There have been many contributors, too many to mention, but I would like to especially thank those who have devoted much time, energy, and encouragement to this project.

My wife, Ann, for proof reading, typing, and re-typing, and re-proofing...

Dr. Judith Burdan, for the final edit of the manuscript;

Margaret Cherry, my mother-in-law, for listening to my stories and laughing at some that weren't really that funny;

The Reverends Paul Coleman, Ron Heffield, and James L. Snyder, for guidance and constructive criticism;

Clarice Sellers, my most fervent cheerleader;

Peggy Ward, for your red pencil and helpful suggestions;

and Rev. Dale Proffitt, who showed me that this IS a book you can put down.

FOREWORD

You are about to embark on a journey, one that will take you into the mind and life of a man born blind. This journey will amuse and entertain you, as well as sadden and enlighten you. It will take you to life in the back hills of rural Indiana, with all the fun and challenges of living in a large family. You will travel to school, not on a big yellow bus, but sometimes on a Greyhound.

This journey will take you on to college where Sam and I met. Despite our initial (and mutual) dislike for each other, God had a plan for us to serve Him together for a lifetime. It was Sam's sense of humor and storytelling abilities that God used to change my opinion of him. Since we were poor college students, we would often just sit for hours and talk. That's where I first heard many of these stories. Most still bring a smile to my heart; others make it break. Some deal specifically with situations experienced as a result of his blindness, but many do not, and are just part of a "normal" life. They all make me realize, however, what a special man God is making Sam into. As you read this book, I think you'll understand why.

Storytelling is in Sam's blood. His grandfather proudly reigned in the "Liar's Chair" at the local store where friends and neighbors would gather to hear the "tall tales" he and others would share. I know this had a big influence on Sam's life, as did his mom and a special teacher from the Indiana School for the Blind whose instruction helped enhance those storytelling skills.

As we have told people about this book, some have not liked the title, *Laughing in the Dark*, but I think it is inspired and appropriate. Many of the stories Sam shares in the following pages are humorous and will make you laugh, and Sam happens to be blind, something we sighted people often associate with darkness. But more than that, the title and the pages that follow reveal what God has done in the heart of a little boy with a dark and broken spirit when Jesus, the Light of the world, gave him a good dose of medicine. Are you ready for yours?

Ann Thompson

PROLOGUE

During the 34 years that my wife Ann and I have been married, I have shared countless stories from my child and adulthood that have made her laugh. "You should write a book!" she has often said. Over the years, her suggestions have slowly become more insistent. Those of you who are married know how "suggestions" gradually begin to sound more like orders and proceed from there to, dare I say it, nagging? Well, my wife has not yet resorted to nagging (she seldom does), and since I adore her, I am writing this book.

Ann is truly a fantastic helpmeet. God has greatly blessed me with a loving, caring, and generous wife. Anything I say about her in the following pages that may appear to indicate otherwise is not intentional. This also goes without saying concerning others I will mention. I have, however, changed names of individuals for two reasons. First, I do not wish to embarrass anyone by my recollections, and second, I do not wish to be sued. Any similarities between those people I mention and those I actually know is purely *intentional*. If any of you recognize yourself, it is my hope that you will laugh along with me. The events which I recall in the following pages have brought me more than a little joy over the six decades of my life, and, upon the suggestions of my wife I am sharing them with you. You must want to laugh; you bought the book.

Life has not always been funny, or fun. At times, it has been painful. I grew up in a situation where one was not laughed with but laughed at. Adults and peers alike were condescending and intimidating. One learned to survive by bullying and intimidating others.

I do not remember laughing much as a child. Since I could not see, I saw nothing worth laughing at. I felt that I was God's big joke. I took life quite seriously. If I laughed, it was often to cover up some insecurity. My laughter was not heart-felt; it was what I was supposed to do in a given situation. Funny things happened around me, but for me, it was like watching a comedy in a different language. People were laughing, and I didn't quite know why.

Then at the age of twenty-one the light came on, the curtain went up, and I began to see the humor around me for the first time. What made the difference? Simply stated--Christ. As I yielded my life to Him, I had a sense of being set free from bondage. I began to realize that I had been taking life too seriously. Funny things had been happening all around me, and I had been missing them. I began to really laugh for the first time in my life. I began to laugh at myself. I began to laugh with, not at, other people. I even discovered that things, funny things, had happened to me because I am blind. I want to share some of them with you.

If you are going to enjoy this book, you must pack up your sensitivity and put it away. I promise you a light-hearted look at blindness, which will, if you let it, seem heartless. Remember this--the author is blind. If I can laugh at silly blunders and stupid mistakes, you should be able to also. So, sit back and enjoy. If I can make you smile for just awhile, the effort is worth it.

Sam Thompson

CONTENTS

Dedication   5
Acknowledgements   6
Foreword   7
Prologue   9
1. Meet The Family   13
2. Hollow Moments   19
3. Family Secrets   37
4. The Things That Happen In Church   41
5. Bathroom Humor   45
6. Getting Around   51
7. Money Talks   63
8. Boy, Could My Mom Cook!   67
9. Animal Stories   71
10. School Days   87
11. Nothing To Laugh About   103
12. Love Is Blind And Kind Of Stupid   113
13. The Eyes Have It   133
14. Some Final Thoughts About My Parents   137

Epilogue   141

CHAPTER 1

Meet the Family

Before I actually start writing in earnest, I think you should meet my family. When all was said and done, there were eleven children. I was number eight. I have been asked why there were so many children in our family. "Well," I've said, "it was cold in the winter, and we did not have television. Mom and Dad had to find something to do." In truth, Mom always wanted a large family. She got it!

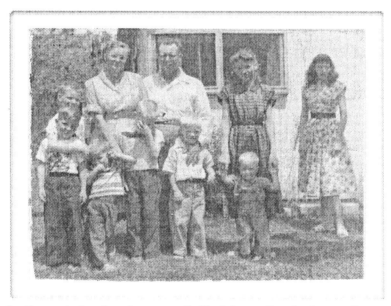

Left to right, back row - Bill, Mom, Dad, Jane, Susan
front row - Jerry, me, Aeris, Mike, Dale
(Dan is MIA, Rick and Tim, not yet born)

Mom and Dad were both previously married. Mom had one daughter, Jane, and Dad had two children, Susan and Dan.

SUSAN: Susan was a curious, nervous, and emotional child. She had a habit of saying what she thought and then thinking about what she had just said. She spent a lot of her life rebuilding bridges she had burned. The funniest story about Susan actually happened before I was born. My parents told the story often, and every time they did in Susan's presence, she would remind them that it was not funny, as they and everyone around them were laughing. Every couple of years, the Ohio River would flood due to excessive rain. For some reason, people would rebuild their homes, live there a couple of years, and then the flood would wipe them out, sometimes taking lives along with property. On one of those flood occasions, Mom and Dad loaded up the family in the old Nash Rambler wagon and made their pilgrimage to the Ohio River to look at the damage. They sat at the edge of the water watching houses, cars, personal household items, and furniture go by. Susan watched intently for a while and then looked at Mom and Dad. "If I find a man in the water, can I keep him?" she asked.

Susan passed away of congestive heart failure in 1998.

JANE: Jane was always quiet and reserved. She would always read to us younger children. She could tell the most delightful stories! My first memory is of Jane holding me. The funniest memory I have of Jane is not one that I actually recall, but one of which I have been told. Jane was always fascinated with cooking. On the occasion of her first apple pie, she excitedly brought it to the table. As she proudly handed Dad the first slice, he reached under his chair and produced a hammer and coal chisel. Jane was not amused, but she was able to laugh about it several years later.

BILL and DAN: Bill and Dan are the same age, and were inseparable as they grew up. They were partners in crime. It seemed like Bill was the one who thought up the mischief and Dan was the one that got caught doing it. My funniest memory of the two of them involves a game of Cowboys and Indians played in the woods that surrounded our house. It seems that the Indians, Dan and Bill, captured one of the Cowboys, my brother Jerry. They tied him to a tree and piled up the wood to burn him at the stake. It was then that Mom's voice could be heard calling, "Supper!"

During the meal Mom looked up from her plate and asked, "Where's Jerry?" "We'll go see if we can find him," Bill and Dan said as they hurried from the table, feigning concern. They went into the woods, untied Jerry, and threatened him within an inch of his life if he told Mom what had happened. Jerry came to the table claiming that he had not heard Mom call.

Bill passed away in 2012 after years of illness.

AERIS: Aeris was both blind and retarded. At least, that was the diagnosis of the doctors when he was young. I personally believe that he had Autism. Once, when Mom would not give Aeris something he wanted, he went into his typical crying and kicking fit. Mom's customary way of dealing with these tantrums was to ignore them. They would usually cease, and things would get back to normal. On this particular day, this routine was followed with apparent success until Aeris walked up behind Mom who was standing at the kitchen stove preparing a meal, grabbed her around the legs just below the knees, picked her up and carried her across the room, putting her down beside his favorite chair. I should point out that he was only about eight years old at the time. From the age of nine, Aeris lived in the Indiana state institutional or residential system.

Aeris passed away in 2013. He always had a favorite chair throughout his lifetime.

JERRY: Jerry was another one of the family who stayed pretty much to himself. Who could blame him? It was dangerous playing with his older brothers. When he was a child, his passion was catching pigeons from a neighbor's barn and trying to make pets out of them, without much success.

MIKE: Mike was the con artist of the family. He could talk anybody out of, or into, just about anything. When you played any game with Mike, you would need to look for new and innovative ways of cheating. When I got older, we would play Monopoly. I never won.

Mike was killed in an auto accident in 1999.

DALE: Dale was the cute one. In fact, he was so cute that no one would believe that our "little angel" could do anything wrong. I will tell you that our little angel's halo was actually two horns that tended to lean towards each other. When Dale would get caught doing something worthy of a spanking, Mom would prepare to administer the punishment. Dale would often look up at her with puppy dog eyes and say, "I love you." Somehow Mom could not spank him when he did that. One day, I thought I would try that gimmick. I deliberately did something wrong and called Mom's attention to it. She brought the sycamore switch and ordered me to "assume the position." I looked up at her with the best puppy dog eyes I could imagine and said those three words, "I love you." Apparently, my eyes were not puppy doggish enough.

RICK: I was eight when Rick was born. The poor guy had to learn how to survive early. As a result, he learned what I call "creative play." Once, when Rick was about two years old, Mike heard him laughing just outside the kitchen door. Mike opened the door to see what was going on and what was so funny. He found Rick on the back step, pencil in hand. "What are you doing?" Mike asked. Rick looked up at him with complete joy in his eyes. "Payin'," he said. Mike stepped out to see what was bringing Rick such joy. There was an old water cistern under that step, which was no longer used since the landlord had dug a well. No one paid much attention to it until that particular day. Due to neglect, a crack had formed between the top of the cistern and the bottom of the step. Rick lay on his belly, looking into that crack. As Mike watched, a copperhead snake stuck its head out of the crack. Rick would jab the snake in the head, and it would retreat back into the darkness below the step. Rick would laugh hysterically. Mike snatched Rick up, amidst much protest, and rushed him into the house. My parents found a nest of snakes in that old cistern. They were killed and the crack was repaired.

TIM: Tim is the baby of the family. He was seven years old when we moved to Florida. One evening shortly after we had relocated, Tim was playing quietly in the front yard. Suddenly we heard a blood-curdling scream, which could only mean disaster. When Mom went to see what Tim was so afraid of, he was standing transfixed in the middle of the yard, trembling uncontrollably. "What is wrong?" Mom asked. Tim finally got his voice back and answered shakily, "I just saw a huge mouse with a shell on its back!" At that moment a large armadillo stuck its head around a tree, obviously as frightened of Tim as he was of it.

Finally, I want you to meet Dad and Mom. After all, they are the reason this family exists.

DAD: Although Dad was quick to become angry and slow to cool down, there were times when he would display his sense of humor. One of those times was when I was either two or three years old. We were listening to the old, battery-powered, floor model Philco radio in our living room. I was fascinated with it, believing that when my family said they heard someone on the radio they were literally "on the radio." I would often walk up to it and try to find who was singing. They kept hiding from me! On one particular occasion, I told Dad that I wanted to sing on the radio. He picked me up and placed me on top of the unit. "Sing," he said. I spent months telling anyone who would listen that I had sung on the radio.

MOM: While Mom was a hard worker, she always seemed to find humor in almost any situation. She was creative and would do what she could to ensure that we enjoyed life. One night, she noticed that we kids were becoming bored with family Bible time. She spent most of the next couple of days locked away in the shed in the back yard. When she emerged, she carried marionettes, which she had whittled by hand and joined together using a complicated system of strings for the joints. She also carried a wooden stage. That evening she told the story of the ten plagues of Egypt. The family still laughs at Pharaoh plagued with lice, jumping wildly all over the stage.

Dad passed away in 1984, Mom in 2000.

You have now met my family. This should assist you when their names are mentioned throughout the book to picture in your mind these individual characters that influenced my life.

By the way, I showed Dale a partial manuscript of this book. He said that he thought I should add a disclaimer stating that my memories are clouded by my old age. I told him he could always write his own book as a rebuttal of what I have written. He smiled mischievously at me and said, "No, I will just wait until the royalties from your book start pouring in, and then I will sue you." He was joking... I hope. Just in case he was not, I think it is in order to tell you that this book would make a great gift for any occasion. Why not purchase several copies for all of your friends and family? I, and my lawyer, will appreciate it.

CHAPTER 2

HOLLOW MOMENTS

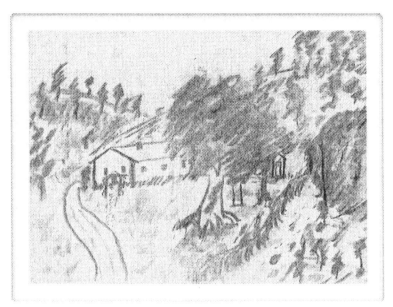

Drawing of The Hollow by Mom, Nona Jane Thompson

When my life began, my family lived in a place that we still affectionately refer to as The Hollow. It was a 30-acre bowl-shaped piece of land. Twenty of the acres were hillside. The original home, located at the bottom of the bowl, burned down when I was an infant. My dad rebuilt a house for us without any plans (an important fact for later stories). This left enough land for farming and lots of mischief. A creek ran just outside the boy's bedroom window. Memories of falling asleep at night with the sound of water running over the stones in the creek bed are still quite vivid.

To most people, The Hollow was just an old run-down farm with a rickety house, inaccessible to the outside world unless one wanted to risk his or her neck to get in. To us, those hills were a wonderland, the house a palace, and the lack of accessibility something that brought our family closer together than we have ever been since.

HOME

When we lived in The Hollow, our family consisted of seven boys and two girls, plus Mom and Dad. All of us were crammed into a house that measured less than a thousand square feet. The girls had a room, a renovated pantry (Dad had forgotten to include a room for them when he rebuilt the house), Mom and Dad had a room that backed up to the chimney flue, and all seven of us boys shared an eight by ten room as far away from the wood stove as you could get and remain in the house. Six of us crammed into one bed, the oldest getting the head of the bed, and Aeris, who would not let anyone sleep with him, got a rollaway bed by himself. Being the next to the youngest at bedtime was not any fun. For the first six years of my life, I slept dodging flailing feet and the aim of the occasional bed wetter. The first night I spent in a bed of my own at the school for the blind, I cried myself to sleep because I was not used to having that much room. I was lonely.

All of the rooms were small with the exception of the kitchen. It was huge! It was large enough to contain all of the usual kitchen equipment—a gas stove, an icebox (until we got electricity, then upgraded to a refrigerator), dishpan, water bucket, and a table that would seat up to twenty. We often had guests in our home, and Mom was able to stretch our meager fair to feed as many as necessary. Needless to say, we were like a lot of large ants in a small anthill. It was for this reason that we did most things outside, including bathing in the summer. More about that later.

I DIDN'T WANT THIS BABY!

The way he came into the world hinted that he was going to be trouble! The "he" I am referring to is my brother Dale. We lived twenty-three miles from town, and he couldn't even wait for Dad to get Mom to the hospital. Dad delivered him in my parent's bedroom on a hot July 4th in 1955. As I heard those first cries, I knew that life had changed forever. Although I was only two, I recognized the fact that my status in life had suddenly changed. I was no longer the baby! I had suddenly, without explanation, been demoted to the position of second in command. As Dad placed the after effects of the delivery into the heating stove to quickly burn them before my older brothers and sisters could get a hold of them, I asked him if he would put the baby in there also. He was not amused. After a hurried trip to the hospital, followed by their return home in a few days with this new baby, I became reconciled to the fact that this "thing" was here to stay, so I might as well get used to it. He was not so bad, at least until he began to walk and talk. It was then that the monster came alive. The problem with this monster was that he was cute, cuddly, and had Mom and Dad wrapped around his little finger. At least, that was the way I saw it. He really wasn't so bad, but he had dethroned me, and I did not like that. He got *my* high chair, *my* potty chair, *my* bed, and more importantly, that special place on *my* Mom's lap. When things went bump in the night and I woke up frightened, my sister came to see what was the matter, not my Mom.

Then one day, I don't know exactly when, I woke up and realized that this little guy was not so bad after all! Yes, he was trouble. Yes, he got me into lots of trouble, but he was really quite okay. There were times when we competed for position, but most of the time we were partners in crime and punishment.

Dale will appear often in future chapters in this book. The truth is that even though I didn't want that baby when he first showed up, he became, and still is, a vital part of my life. Dale was the one who would drop his plans when I came home for the weekend from the school for the blind. Dale was the one who discovered, even before I did, that I might not have any idea what certain things really looked like and saw to it that I could actually touch some of them. He still does this today.

The writer of Proverbs tells us "there is a friend that sticks closer than a brother" (18:24). How great God's love and friendship must be towards us! Honestly, I cannot imagine a relationship with a brother that could be closer than the one Dale and I had when we were growing up. We are still close. If it is possible to be even closer to God, then this motivates me to continue to keep the doors open to that close relationship.

DALE'S PACKRAT HOLE

For those of you who do not know, a packrat is a rodent that will steal anything it can carry, taking it back to its nest and hiding it. Packrats are especially attracted to shiny things and food, not unlike Dale. It seems that as soon as he started walking, he discovered that Susan and Jane would spend some of the money they earned from babysitting and other jobs on candy and stash it in their room, off limits to the boys. I do not recall how Dale discovered the stash since we were not permitted in their room. All I do remember is that the girls began to notice that candy, jewelry, and coins were missing.

When Dad built the house, he, for some unexplainable reason, left a cubbyhole about two feet square just above the baseboard on the left wall of the hallway that ran back to the girls' room. Remember, their room was originally designed as a pantry, but the girls had taken it over. This cubbyhole was where Dale would stash his booty after lifting it from the girls' room. Mom discovered this hiding place while cleaning the house one day. I happened to be playing near her when she did so and took note of the place. My plan was a great one! Dale would steal the candy, hide it in his hole, and I would steal the candy from Dale. Now that he was caught, he would get into trouble, and I would enjoy the rare candy bar without any consequences. This plan worked quite well for some time until I came upon Dale in the hallway one afternoon. Rather than taking the time to go outside to the outhouse, he was taking care of business in his packrat hole. Even at the age of four, I lost all appetite for candy from that particular hiding place.

TOOLS OF THE TRADE

There were three times in my childhood that Dale and Dad's tools came together to make a lasting impression on my life, not to mention my backside. When I was quite young, it was our family custom that we all rise early, perform our various chores, and then gather around the big table in the kitchen for a hearty Midwestern breakfast before Dad went off to work. Before Dale came along, this was my time with Dad. I would sit in my highchair next to him, and we would talk and play while we ate. This changed after Dale was big enough to sit at the table. I was moved down to the other end of the table next to my sister Jane, and Dale was placed in *my* chair and sat in *my* spot. Dad played and talked with *him*. To say I did not like this arrangement is an understatement.

One morning while Dad was playing and talking with Dale, and while Mom was dealing with all of the typical calamities and conflicts of a large family getting started in the morning, I slipped out the back door, across the backyard, past the outhouse, and into Dad's tool shed. After all, no one was paying attention to me, and I had always been fascinated with the chainsaw. I liked the noise it made and would often be caught messing with it. For obvious reasons, I had plenty of opportunities to ponder the pain in my backside for trying to get the saw started. I do not know how it happened this particular morning. Somehow, I got the saw started! I jumped away from it and ran into the house, screaming in terror. Dad had already heard the noise and passed me on his way to the shed. When he returned, I finally had some time with Dad. He talked, he spanked, but he didn't play. Dale was oblivious to the trouble he had caused. He just sat there in *my* chair contentedly eating his biscuits and gravy, chattering happily to anyone who would listen.

The second time involved a brand new, not even out of the box, soldering iron of Dad's. A two-year-old Dale brought it to a four-year-old me and informed me that it needed fixed. "Daddy told me that he wants you to fix it," he told me. He had also brought me a hammer out of Dad's toolbox. I removed the iron from its box, placed it on the wooden step just outside the back door of our house, and proceeded to "fix" it by pounding it to smithereens! When Dad got home that evening, I proudly displayed my "repair" job. Need I say that he was not happy? Dale claimed no knowledge of the whole event. Imagine that!

Needless to say, Dad was very protective of his tools and for good reason. Several of my older brothers would "borrow" Dad's tools, lose or break them, or simply not return them. When Dad discovered this, he would rant and rave until the guilty party confessed. That party would then be, metaphorically speaking, taken to the woodshed, and life would return to normal. This was the way things happened until Dale devised a scheme that would eventually get me into more trouble than I could imagine.

It had been awhile since Dad had yelled about any missing or broken tools. My brothers had learned their lesson and only used tools after receiving permission. Then one day, Dad started yelling again. Tools had begun to systematically disappear once again. None of the older boys knew anything about them. They would not even confess after trips to the woodshed. "Maybe Sammy took them," Dale offered. "Sammy would not take my tools," Dad replied. And I wouldn't have. But that all changed.

One day, shortly after the last tool disappeared and Dad had unsuccessfully interrogated my older brothers, Dale took me into his confidence. He led me out into the shallow creek that ran through the yard beside our house, removed a large rock from over a hole he had dug in the center of it and displayed several rusty tools that he had been hiding there for the past several months. We had a good laugh. He had really pulled one over on Dad!

"Why don't you take a tool and hide it here?" he asked innocently. "I won't tell on you." I actually believed him. I asked him to keep Dad busy while I went to the shed to get a tool. He agreed. That was a big mistake.

I slipped around the house, across the back yard, past the outhouse and into Dad's tool shed. Dad had a huge Farm All Tractor. This old relic was one of those tractors with the huge crank that you placed in the side of the motor. You adjusted the gas mixture and the spark, turned the crank until the motor fired and jumped back before the crank kicked and broke your arm. The crank would spin wildly until it finally fell out. Attachments were changed and repairs were made using a large wrench designed for that particular model of tractor. Not realizing that the hole Dale had dug would not hold it, I lugged that wrench out of the tool shed and headed for the creek.

In the meantime, Dale had kept Dad busy by informing him that I had told him about my caper of stealing his tools and hiding them in the creek. I slipped quietly down the creek bank, listened for any signs that I had been detected, and waded to the rock. I placed the wrench on the wet rocky bottom of the creek and picked up the rock. It was then that I felt two large hands on my shoulders and, soon, another painful impression on my backside.

SLIPPIN' AND SLIDIN'

Across the creek from the house was, what I perceived as a child to be, a high clay cliff. In actuality, it was probably no more than twenty feet high, if that. In the summer, we would spend hours each day playing on this cliff. One of our favorite things to do was to dig "caves" in the side of it. Each cave could hold a couple of boys. They would last until we got a good rain, and then they would wash out. Mom helped us build a couple of caves that lasted through several rainstorms. She seemed to know how to do lots of neat things, like digging caves that would last.

Mom was a very specific disciplinarian. She would tell us in no uncertain terms what she expected of us, and we knew that we should do exactly what she said or face the consequences. When Mom told Dale and me that we were not to slide down the cliff into the creek on flattened out cardboard boxes, we stopped doing it. We simply slid down the cliff into the creek on the seats of our pants. Needless to say, Mom was not happy with our interpretation of her instructions, yet she could not punish us because we were no longer sliding down the cliff into the creek on flattened out cardboard boxes.

Another favorite past time was to swing on wild grape vines over the various gullies found in The Hollow. My older brothers especially liked partially cutting a vine so that when our sisters would swing out over a gully, the vine would break, and the girls would end up in a tree, or at the bottom of the gully. This happened to me a couple of times, and then I wised up. I would not swing on a vine unless one of the older boys did it first.

When snow fell, the hills around the house would be instantly transformed into a winter playground to suit any child's dream. There were sledding hills for anyone with just about any level of expertise. There were small hills for the younger, and huge, steep hills for the older and less faint of heart. The problem was that we never owned a sled while we lived in The Hollow. This lack necessitated creativity. Until Mom stopped us, we would take the knob off the lid of her round Maytag wringer type washer and slide down the hills on that lid. One person could sit on the lid and fly down a hill, turning round and round at breakneck speed. After Mom put a stop to this sled, my two oldest brothers discovered an even greater one.

Dad had an old International pickup truck. The thing was used for just about everything. When the old Plymouth was not running, it became the family's sole means of transportation. It was used to haul things around the property, as well as moving gravel from the creek bed to the lane so that it could be negotiated by cars. In the winter, the truck was parked down by the house, while the car was left up on the road. No one wanted to attempt to get a vehicle down the hill in the winter unless it was totally necessary. Dad always figured that the truck was the vehicle most likely to make it up the hill if we ever had an emergency mandating the need for transportation.

For the most part, the truck was ignored during the winter. My brothers discovered that the hood made an excellent sled. It could be removed and replaced quickly, at least two people could ride on it, and it was fast! For two or three weeks, they would wait for Mom and Dad to leave, skip school, take the hood off the truck, and spend the day sledding. They would stop in time to remount the hood, walk up and down the hill to leave tracks, and bribe or threaten my sisters. This plan worked fine until the day Dan ran into a tree. That wreck really messed up the hood! The boys tried to remount it onto the truck, but it was so deformed, it would not close. They decided to leave it, hoping that Dad would not notice. He noticed!

A LITTLE PRIVACY, PLEASE?

In the summer, Mom would often hand us boys a bar of soap and a washcloth on Saturday afternoon and send us out into the creek to take a bath. The girls got the privilege of bathing in the back yard in the galvanized steel washtub that had been filled with water from the well in the morning and left out in the sun to warm up.

One Saturday that I remember well started as usual. Knowing that it was bath day, the older boys scattered into the woods. They would have to be found and dragged home kicking and screaming for their baths. Dale and I had not quite gotten into that strategy yet, so Mom handed us our equipment and shooed us like chickens into the yard for our Saturday ritual.

There were only two people besides Mom and Dad who would drive down the hill into The Hollow at that time—my uncle Bob and the Preacher. Later, the man who owned the grocery store twelve miles away would get up the nerve to drive down in his huckster wagon, but that is another story.

On this particular day, Dale and I were reluctantly taking our baths when the Preacher and his wife pulled up right in front of us. We both tried to hide in the few inches of water on the bottom of the creek, but the laughter of the Preacher's wife convinced us that it was doing no good. Dale and I jumped out of the creek, and each of us ran dripping to our hiding places. I don't remember where Dale went, but I locked myself in the outhouse. It didn't take long before I got tired of that smelly place. I began crying, and Mom, Dad, the Preacher and his wife kept encouraging me to come out. I wouldn't. About ten minutes after they left, I was coaxed into the house. Mom could never get me back into that creek again for a bath. I got the privilege of bathing in the tub in the backyard. But that, too, had its problems.

Occasionally military jets would fly overhead on their return from the bombing range that was not far from us. I became convinced that people in those planes could see me if I was in the tub in the backyard. Mom finally persuaded me otherwise, and through the entire summer, I bathed without any problem until the last Saturday of August. I remember that it was the last Saturday because Mom said that was going to be the last week we bathed outside for that year. We always started taking our Saturday night baths inside after Labor Day.

I was in the tub, bathing like a good boy, when a jet flew over. I paid no attention to it. After all, Mom told me that I could not be seen. One of my brothers had a plan that would shake my faith in Mom's word for quite some time. He hid in a nearby tree, and when the plane flew over, he whistled. I was out of that tub in a millisecond and in the house. It took years for me to figure out what had happened. Mom had a difficult time getting me to take a bath after that.

While I would not bathe in the creek, I would still play in it. Even though our yard was shaded by big oak trees and stayed pretty cool during the heat of the day, there is something about a gently running creek that says to a young and mischievous boy, "Come in. Get wet!" Dale and I were particularly capable of hearing that call. We played in the creek for hours at a time. When our pants got wet, we would simply cast them, along with the underwear, onto the creek bank and continue playing until Mom caught us and made us put on dry clothes. We fussed and complained, but in the end Mom would win and we would be fully clothed and out the door again. In a short time, Mom was dragging us back inside for another dressing. We liked the water, but we did not like wet clothes. It was my passionate dislike of wet pants that eventually embarrassed my sister Jane to the point that she still blushes when the following story comes up in family conversations.

My parents did not take the family out much. Maybe it was because there were so many of us, or maybe (and I believe this was the real reason) we were such an embarrassment to them. Once a year, however, we did go to an amusement park in Indianapolis. Riverside Amusement Park was a kid's dream! It was one of those old parks with old-fashioned rides like wooden roller coasters, a big wooden carousel, and other rides that, when you mention them, looks of nostalgia cross faces of those who remember. The focal point of the park for teenagers was the "Tunnel of Love". Passengers would board a wooden boat that meandered through what seemed like an endless tunnel for a three-year-old who was forced to go on this ride by an older sister. Granted, Jane would have probably preferred another partner besides her younger brother, but, since she had been given charge of me, and since she wanted to go, I went along.

There was a surprise at the end of the ride, however. The boat would slowly begin ascending a ramp. At the top it would burst out into bright sunlight, catching young lovers in all kinds of embraces. Before they could catch their breath and gather their wits, the boat plunged down another ramp, back into the water, soaking everyone aboard. Jane and I were in the back of the boat, so we got especially wet! I finally enjoyed that ride.

As soon as we got off the boat, Jane ran into my other sister, Susan, who was accompanied by some of their mutual friends. I stood quietly as they knotted together to talk about whatever it was that girls could find to talk about. As I stood there, those wet pants began to bother me. I did what came naturally. I proceeded to go "au naturel." Jane did not notice until she heard giggles and people started pointing. Susan skedaddled, leaving Jane with the task of putting pants back on a protesting three-year-old. She held me over one arm while, with the other, she tried to catch my kicking feet as I screamed, "I want them off! I want them off!" I don't remember Jane spanking me, or even raising her voice at me, but I do remember wearing wet pants the rest of the day.

BE CAREFUL WHAT YOU ASK FOR!

On warm summer days, Dad used to sit out under the big oak tree next to the creek, chew his tobacco, and spit the juice into the running water beside him. The particular tobacco he chewed had a wonderful wintergreen scent. Dale and I were intrigued by that scent and used to beg Dad to let us try some of that tobacco for ourselves. He always said no, until one day when he held out the can for us. "Take as much as you like," he said.

This was the moment we had waited for! We each dug our grubby hands into that can, placed the large portion into our eager mouths, and swallowed the mouthful. Can you say FIRE? Our first and immediate reaction was to run to the well for water, which, coincidently, made that tobacco swell up inside our tummies. All I remember after that was lying on the creek bank heaving up food I had not even eaten yet, hanging onto the grass to keep from falling off of the world. Dad was literally rolling on the ground, laughing himself to tears. Mom, on the other hand, was not too happy with him. Needless to say, I did not chew tobacco when I got older.

THE HUCKSTER WAGON

In the days of the early pioneers it was normal for families not to have neighbors nearby. The nearest settlement could be miles away, making it difficult for some families to acquire basic staples they might need to run a household. The owner of the "local" general store would often load a wagon with basic supplies and head for distant homesteads. This huckster wagon was a welcome sight as it approached these lonely families.

It was in that spirit that the owner of the local general store acquired an old school bus. He removed all of the seats, with the exception of the driver's seat, of course, and replaced them with shelves. Since it was difficult for most families to get to the store on a regular basis, he came to the families. He was one of the few who would tackle the steep driveway into The Hollow. Wanting the money he could possibly receive from servicing our large family, he bolted the shelves to the floor, rigged straps to keep the merchandise on the shelves, and headed down the hill.

Tuesday evening was Huckster Wagon Night. I looked forward to hearing the echo of the bus horn through the trees as it began the descent into The Hollow. I would run for my few pennies or my returnable pop bottles. It did not matter if I had one pop bottle, a nickel or a quarter; I could get anything I wanted off that bus for whatever I had. It sure made it hard for Mom and Dad to teach me the value of money. I honestly thought you could buy anything for a penny.

MOVING OUT

My family moved in and out of The Hollow several times when I was a child. We moved out for the last time when I was nine years old. That day began early for me. For some reason, I was up before dawn, sitting on the front step. My nine-year-old mind was remembering the happy times that we as a family had experienced in the house and in the woods surrounding it. I sat listening to the creek murmuring off to my left and remembered many of the things I have shared with you and some others I have not. I felt the cool Fall air on my cheek. As I sat there, the sun began to rise. It would be quite some time before one would feel the effects of that sunrise in The Hollow, but the animals knew. It was as though a switch was thrown. All of the night sounds ceased, and the day began with the song of one solitary bird somewhere in the woods, up the hill and to my left. And then I felt it—the mist of morning.

I sat there for what seemed to be hours. I felt the cool of the night give way to the warmth of the day. I could see the sunlight peeking through the trees (I had light perception at the time). That memory stamped indelibly on my mind has brought me much comfort in my adult life. When I think of how my life was before Christ entered into it, I remember the cool night air. But when Christ came into my life, the night ceased, light and warmth came, and the past became a distant memory. Just as I was able to get up off that front step and follow my family to the next dwelling place, knowing that somehow everything was going to be all right, I, after Christ came into my life, was able to follow Him, knowing that everything *was* all right.

From time to time, various family members went back to visit The Hollow. They would stand at the top of the hill and remember the outhouse that Dad put there so that the kids did not have to wait in the cold for the school bus. They would laugh at the memory of Jane and Susan freezing because they were not about to wait inside that building until the bus came because they did not want their friends laughing at them. They would remember carrying wood down from the hillside for heating the little house during the cold winters. They would remember becoming fond of animals that we later ate. They would laugh at the memory of my brother Jerry sitting on the roof of the house, holding the television antenna so that Dad could watch *Bonanza* on Sunday nights. It seemed that those hills rang with memories that only the Thompson family could hear, but we always heard them clearly.

On December 27, 2003, Dale and I, along with our families, found and hiked down into The Hollow. As I stepped out of the car and started toward the top of the hill, memories rushed back. Once again, I was a child rambling through those woods. I could almost hear Mom calling us in for a meal. I could almost smell the homemade bread and taste the fresh vegetables that came from our garden. I could almost hear the panther Mom had fed screaming somewhere in those woods.

As we got down to the level clearing where the house and out buildings stood, we discovered that there was not much left. The house had fallen, and only one partial wall and the chimney remained standing. The old oak tree is now about ten feet in diameter and about ninety feet high. Grape vines that we used to swing on were as big around as my arm.

Dale and I spent several minutes remembering. We found old familiar spots and laughed at forgotten memories, memories that flooded back into our minds. We laughed about locking Santa Claus (Dad) out of the house one Christmas and about how angry he had become as he was unable to get in out of the cold. We laughed when we remembered Santa's language that Christmas morning. We remembered the rope breaking as Mom lifted the bucket out of the well, and Jerry being lowered down by a rope to retrieve it. We remembered how Mom would sell the television every summer, until Dad discovered *Bonanza*, that is. We remembered how crowded the living room would get when we all wanted to watch television, and how Mom would make popcorn during the summer and pull the television into the front door, and we would sit out in the yard and watch our favorite shows. The memories just kept rushing back.

Finally, it was time to go. As I turned to walk up that big hill to the car, I felt pangs of regret that I could not relive those days. They will, however, continue to live on in my memory, and now, maybe, just maybe, they will come to life for you, too.

CHAPTER 3

FAMILY SECRETS

THE KID IN DAD

Most of the time, Dad did not interact much with us unless there was a need for discipline. At times, however, the kid in him would come out. We boys always looked forward to those events, and took full advantage of them.

One of those regular occasions was our annual trek to Riverside Amusement Park in Indianapolis. The kid really came out in Dad on that day! He made it his purpose to out-ride any of the boys. This usually resulted in Mom driving home because Dad was suffering from extreme motion sickness. One particular year, Dad took my brother Aeris to ride on the Thriller. This wooden roller coaster was one of those fast, bumpy, jerky rides that gave anyone who dared to ride it an instant need for a long-term association with a chiropractor.

Aeris loved this ride! The operator recognized Aeris' disability and permitted him to stay on the ride when it was time to reload. After about the sixth time, Dad was ready to get off. Aeris wanted no part of that! He clung to the bar, even though it was raised, and screamed at the top of his lungs. Dad rode a couple of times more, and, once again, tried to get Aeris off, to no avail. He convinced the operator that Aeris would stay put if he let him ride alone. The operator consented, and Dad went off to the side to lose the lunch he had not yet eaten. After several more rides, Aeris fell asleep. He was easily removed from the ride at that point. Dad gave up his quest to outride the boys that day.

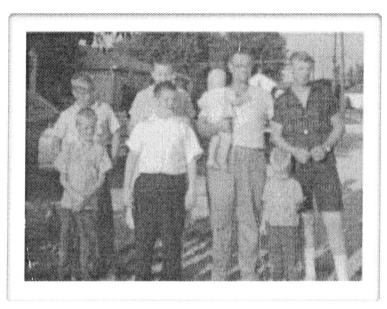
Dad and the boys (without Aeris)

CURIOUS SAM

I was a curious boy. It did not matter what kind of store we were in, or what we were shopping for, I would feel the merchandise on the shelves, trying to discover what was inside. At the age of ten, I was with Mom and Dad in a dollar store while on our way home from school for the weekend. As usual, I was investigating my surroundings when I came upon something totally foreign to me. My hands discovered a neatly stacked display of soft, round, cup-shaped items. I was fascinated with them. Dad sauntered up beside me and asked me if I knew what those things were. When I said no, he informed me in a whisper loud enough for Mom and anyone else in proximity to hear, that they were brassieres (this was not the actual term he used). I moved my hand away like those things were on fire! Mom, Dad, and a few customers laughed loudly. I think my face was red for an hour. Dad loved to tell that story whenever friends and family were visiting. And, by the way, guess what I got for Christmas that year?

DENTURED SERVITUDE

About this same time, Dad was working for the Parks and Recreation Department in the City of Columbus, Indiana. One of his jobs was to maintain the Potter's Field, a cemetery for the poor and indigent. When a plot would get crowded, Dad and a helper would dig up some of the older graves and stack the coffins to make room for more. Dad's partner was not a particularly hard worker. Dad often said that Dick (his real name) did not mind work—he could watch someone do it all day long. While Dad was down in the grave digging, Dick would be sitting under a tree, or standing by the open grave chattering away. He would often sample what Dad had packed for lunch. Since Dick had seniority, Dad could not change partners without jeopardizing his job. He struggled about what to do about Dick until an opportunity presented itself.

Dad had planned on getting dentures for quite some time since he had lost all of his teeth to a gum condition. When he finally had the funds, he was fitted and scheduled to pick up his new teeth on a Saturday morning. He said nothing to his co-workers about this new acquisition and swore all of us to secrecy. He had a plan, and a great one it was!

The Friday before he was to pick up his new teeth, he volunteered Dick and himself to work the Potter's Field on Monday. The supervisor was excited to have willing people to do this task, since he usually had to threaten a team to get them to go.

On that Monday morning, Dad placed his new teeth in the pocket of his coveralls and headed to work, confident that he would have a new partner on Tuesday.

After arriving at the sight, it did not take long for the usual scenario to set up. Dad was in the grave, and Dick was standing at the edge, chattering away as usual. As Dad was digging, he struck the top of a wooden coffin.

Turning his back to Dick, and acting like he was going to pick up the coffin, he said, "Dick, I will need your help." As Dick descended into the grave behind him, Dad reached down toward the coffin with his right hand, while quickly retrieving the teeth from his pocket with his left.

"Look what I found," he said, holding up the dentures. As he turned to face Dick, he opened his mouth wide and put the teeth in place. "They fit! How about that! I needed some new teeth! You never know what you will find."

Dad climbed out of the grave and opened his lunch box and took a big bite out of a sandwich. "I don't want this, Dick. Do you want it?" White as a sheet, Dick declined. He worked especially hard to get the task finished that day. As soon as he and Dad pulled up to the shop that afternoon, Dick requested a new partner.

CHAPTER 4

THE THINGS THAT HAPPEN AT CHURCH!

My family changed churches several times when I was a child. From the stories Mom told me about my actions, I can't help but wonder if I was the reason. Perhaps you can help me decide if this is true as you analyze the following examples of my behavior.

ACCIDENTS WILL HAPPEN!

The church we attended when I was an infant was one of those churches with a lot of character. In other words, it was kind of run down. The pews were old and unleveled. As is typical with babies, I often fell asleep during the service. Since there was no nursery, Mom simply placed me on the pew beside her, and I would sleep soundly for quite some time. This particular morning went as usual until I did what babies also do naturally. I wet my diaper. The problem was that my plastic pants leaked (this was before disposable diapers that keep everything locked inside). The contents of my diaper slowly leaked out around the edges, flowed towards the crevice formed by the meeting of the seat and back. Since the pew was not level, the crevice was a natural channel the liquid could flow down towards the opposite end of the pew from where I was comfortably sleeping. Other than Mom and me, the pew was filled with non-family members who suddenly began to get a warm feeling behind them. It did not take long for them to realize that this feeling was not a result of the preacher's message. They began to squirm, and then some jumped to their feet. All had trouble explaining the wet spots on their backsides as they left. Mom said she got some unusual looks that morning as folks began to figure out what happened, and she ended up sitting alone for several weeks after that.

LEFT ALONE

A few weeks later, I fell fast asleep again during the morning service. When the service was over Mom asked Jane to see that I got to the truck. Jane, in turn, asked Susan. The end result was that no one picked me up. We lived 23 miles from the church. The large Thompson family was loaded into the back of the pickup truck for the ride home. It was so confusing and noisy that Mom did not notice that I was not being carried by anyone. It was a normal occurrence for the older kids to look after the younger, and Mom assumed that this was what had happened and that I had been carried inside and placed in my crib where I was sleeping. Imagine her surprise when she went to check on me after the family had eaten. She and Dad rushed back to town, woke up the pastor from his afternoon nap and found me where they had left me. I was screaming my head off. The pastor looked at them and said, "If you didn't want this one, I am sure that there is someone in the congregation who would not mind a good pet." He smiled and patted my head. It was a big joke around the church for quite some time. For years after that, my nickname was Pet.

THAT'S NOT THE RIGHT SONG!

A couple of years later when I was talking, I was given the privilege of singing "Away in a Manger" in the children's Christmas program. I was so tiny that I could not be seen if I stood behind the rail that surrounded the platform. During rehearsal, the pastor's wife would stand me on the rail and hold me from behind while I belted out my solo with gusto. The night of the program the little church was filled to capacity. My turn came, and I was lifted to my perch where I could be seen. The pianist began playing "Away in a Manger," and I began singing "Up on the housetop reindeer paws..." The place erupted! I was removed from the rail, and it was quite some time before I received any more opportunities to perform at that church.

THE DAY I ALMOST GOT KICKED OUT OF SUNDAY SCHOOL

I had a bad speech impediment until I was about seven years old. Any word that began with a "tr", I would pronounce "fw". With this impediment, the word "tree" would be "fwee." Needless to say, certain words could sound like some other words. This was the case when my dad got a new job hauling asphalt for a local company. I was fascinated with the fact that my dad drove a big truck. I told anyone that would listen that my dad was a big "fwucker."

The morning I announced this fact to my Sunday School teacher, who happened to also be the pastor's wife, was an unforgettable day. I blurted out the news loudly in front of the entire class. Mrs. Brown's shock was evident by the way she quickly ushered me out of the classroom straight to my mother. She insisted that I repeat what I had just said to her in front of the class full of impressionable five year olds. When I repeated the announcement, Mom burst into laughter, which did not help Mrs. Brown's disposition until Mom reminded her of my speech impediment. Needless to say, from then on I was required to tell Mrs. Brown what I wanted to say to the class before I was permitted to say it out loud.

CHAPTER 5

BATHROOM HUMOR

No, it is not what you think! As a blind person, I have had several experiences with bathrooms that are both unusual and amusing. I will relate some of them in this chapter.

I BROKE IT!

We did not have indoor plumbing in our home until after I went away to the school for the blind. In fact, all of our friends and relatives had outhouses. I cannot recall ever being in an indoor bathroom until I used my first one at the school. That was a day I will always remember. I went into the bathroom as instructed and did what comes naturally. After finishing, I began to feel around on the wall out of curiosity. I found the round smooth handle and pulled it. The noise frightened me out of my wits! I ran out of the bathroom, my pants around my ankles, yelling, "I broke it!" The housemother was laughing so hard that it took her a few minutes to explain to me that things were supposed to work like that.

IF ONLY I COULD READ

When I was in the sixth grade, our school band was awarded the opportunity to travel to an amusement park to take part in a band festival. After we performed, we were given ride tickets and turned loose on the park. My "buddy" for the day had some vision but not much. When the "urge" hit us, we headed off for the rest rooms.

We entered the room, and I immediately found a stall. My buddy discovered that he had accidentally directed us into the lady's room. Rather than telling me, he beat a hasty retreat. I wised up when I heard a chorus of high voices as a group of girls from my school entered the restroom. I sat as quietly as I could and waited. When all was silent, I emerged, exiting as quickly as possible. Later on the bus one of the girls with limited vision sat down beside me.

"I thought you were never going to come out of the restroom earlier today," she said.

"What do you mean?"

"I recognized your shoes. I hung around outside the door to see if I was right. I was." Boy, was I embarrassed.

"Don't worry," she said, "it is our little secret."

IN THE LOCK-UP

One of the homes in which we lived was an old, run-down house next to the railroad tracks in Garden City, Indiana. The "facility" for this house was an even more run-down outhouse. When the wind blew, the door would swing back and forth, creaking noisily. Dad fixed that situation by driving a nail through a small piece of a two by four and positioning it so that it could be pivoted across the door from the frame. This would hold the door shut, thus stopping the disturbance.

Next to this old outhouse was a tree, the branches of which hung over the railroad tracks. It did not take Dale and me long to discover that we could climb this tree, and when a train roared by underneath, have quite a wild ride as the vacuum created would pull the branch down toward the top of the train. The turbulence between cars made for a free amusement park ride, one with more than a hint of danger.

One of my Mom's sisters came to stay with us between marriages. She was always high strung. She did not seem to ever be amused by the things that amused Dale and me. One particular morning as Dale and I were in our perch awaiting the morning passenger train, our aunt came to use the outhouse. She noticed us in the tree and announced that she was in a hurry, but if we were not out of that tree when she finished, we would be in a heap of trouble. When she got inside the building and locked the door, I convinced Dale to shimmy down the tree and lock the outside lock. He was more than willing to do so. He got back up the tree just in time. The train whistled at the crossing a few yards down from where we were perched and roared underneath us. Our aunt tried to get out of the door at the same time. We could tell she was screaming, but we could not understand her. While the train was still roaring by, we hurried down the tree and headed for the front yard. She kept yelling, saying things I will not repeat. Dale ran around the side of the house and threw a well-aimed stick at the lock, which caused it to pivot out of the way. He had just barely turned it across the door. Our aunt nearly fell out of the door because she was pushing on it. We stayed away from home the rest of the day.

AN UPSETTING EXPERIENCE

My brothers, Dan and Bill, had an interesting pastime. Around Halloween each year, they would gather up a couple or three of their friends and look for outhouses to upset. They considered it to be especially fun if they could find one that was occupied. No one could quite prove that they were involved in this practice, but everyone in the neighborhood suspected them.

One year, a neighbor who had a reputation for drinking too much and sitting out on his front porch with his shotgun waiting for anyone to drive up "his hill" passed the word around the neighborhood that he would shoot anyone who dared to upset his outhouse on Halloween. That was like saying "sic 'em" to a dog. Dan, Bill, and their friends planned their strategy and anxiously awaited nightfall. When it was pitch dark, they quietly sneaked into our neighbor's back yard. They could see the dim shape of the outhouse in front of them. So far, so good! They lined up side by side, shoulder to shoulder, stretching the entire width of the small wooden building. One of them quietly whispered, "One. Two. Three!" On three, they rushed the building. It had been moved back ten feet. The whole line sunk to their armpits in the waste pit. At that moment, the porch light came on, and they heard the sound of a gunshot. Those boys headed for the nearby lake and jumped in the freezing water, soiled clothes and all.

When they were sure the coast was clear, they headed down the hill to our house. Mom suspected something when she heard the shot and was waiting for them in the backyard, where they headed, planning to do, who knows what, about their clothes! Mom made all of them strip down completely. She turned on the hose and doused all of them with cold spring water. Their howls and exclamations woke up several of the neighbors. Porch lights clicked on all over the place.

"We're cold!" they exclaimed. Mom did not even flinch. "You can warm up by the fire I built to try to burn those nasty clothes." After saying that, she went to call the neighbor boys' parents, asking them to bring them some clothes. Boy, were they humiliated! That was the last year they upset outhouses.

WHERE DID IT GO?

It would often be quite some time between home visits when I was attending school. I left home for the beginning of the school year when I was in the fifth grade and did not return home for a couple of months. I knew that the pit under the family outhouse in the back yard was getting full and that Dad would soon, with the help of my brothers, dig a new one and move the building. I knew he would cover up the old pit and Mom would plant some kind of tree where it had been.

That is exactly what happened. However, when I came home for a weekend visit, no one told me about the relocation of the outhouse. Since it was late when I got home, I simply walked around to the side of the house and took care of business behind a tree before going to find a place to sleep. But, in the middle of the night, I had to go. Boy, did I have to go! I slipped out the back door and up the path. A mound of dirt with a little sprig of a tree greeted me where the outhouse was supposed to be. I spent an hour searching the yard for that outhouse! My stomach kept reminding me that I had better find it soon. I never did. That was a long night! As soon as I heard movement in the kitchen, I was up. I have never been so happy to see an old wooden building in my life!

DEFINITELY NOT A GOOD SITUATION

A few years ago, Ann and I went to meet some out-of-town friends at a local restaurant. Since I, at times, consume equal amounts of food and liquid, I found it necessary to visit the "facility" before departing from the establishment. I hate public restrooms! You never know who, or what, you will find in them. As a blind person, I find it necessary to feel my way around once inside. It was nice when I had my guide dog, Strider (more about him later). I could tell him what I was looking for, and he would find it. This particular night happened after Strider retired. I was on my own!

I trailed along the wall searching for an open stall. That is usually a safe bet. I found one, the handicapped stall. I walked inside and immediately patted a man on the backside. I stepped back, surprised. He swung around with an oath and immediately began to call my mother and me some awful names. I was running around the room, bouncing off fixtures, all the time explaining at the top of my voice that I was blind. He was not listening. I finally got back around the room to the stall he had vacated. I got inside and locked the door. He stood outside of the stall door, shaking it and threatening me loudly. I think he had taken too many trips to the bar. Thankfully, he did not try to come under the door. After a few minutes, it grew quiet. I was not sure if he had left or was just waiting silently for me. I let several men come and go before I worked up the nerve to come out of that stall. The funny thing is, I never used the facility!

CHAPTER 6

GETTING AROUND

Conveyance for a person who is blind can often be a challenge or, at the least, an interesting experience. Over the course of my life, I have had some interesting experiences and have been the cause of some for others.

A DOLLAR A CARLOAD

Drive-in movie theaters were quite popular when I was young. Often, the local drive-in would have special promotions where admission was only a dollar for a carload. Of course, to the management, a carload was the capacity of a car where all passengers were seated comfortably and properly. My brother Bill had a different interpretation, however.

Bill had acquired a 1953 Dodge convertible. He would place a couple of us younger kids in the pocket where the top rested when it was down and partially lower it. He would explain to the ticket taker that his top was broken and that he could not get it to move either way. Two or three more of us would be in the trunk. The back floorboard held a couple, and both the front and rear seats were filled to capacity. As soon as the dollar was paid and the car was parked inside, we would all pile out and find speakers in the adjacent parking spots. Needless to say, management did not like our arrangement and took to searching Bill's car before he was admitted.

Since the Dodge was declared off limits, Bill "borrowed" Dad's International three-quarter ton flatbed truck. About twenty of us piled on and we headed for the drive-in. We were not permitted in for a dollar because management said that the truck was not a car. Imagine that!

EVERYBODY ON THE BUS!

When I entered the fourth grade, Mom and Dad decided I was old enough to ride the bus home for weekends. This made it possible for me to leave the school a little more often since they did not need to take off work to come and get me. Since Dad was frequently out of work and needed to find new work someplace else, I would often receive a bus ticket in the mail from my parents, but they would not tell me that we had moved. There would simply be an envelope enclosed with the words "Cab Driver" on it. After arriving in my hometown, I would ask the station attendant to call me a cab, hand the driver the envelope, and exit the cab when he pulled up to the house. Mom and Dad never locked the doors to any home, so I would simply find the door on my own, if the driver did not offer to assist me, go inside, and acquaint myself with my new surroundings. Quite an adventure!

Since a number of students from the school rode public transportation to their homes, bus drivers got comfortable with our presence and would do what they could to make our trips as easy as possible since we often traveled alone. They got so comfortable, in fact, that some would play little practical jokes on us. On my first trip to Columbus as a small boy, I experienced one of those drivers.

A Traveler's Aid representative would take me to the bus and see that I was seated. As we got to the bus, the driver told me that I could go ahead and board and he would get my ticket later. There were a number of people behind me, and he wanted the representative to be able to get off the bus without difficulty. I got seated, and, as he promised, he came back, stubbed my ticket, started the bus, and away we went.

I was seated right behind him, so he glanced back and asked, "Where are you getting off?"

"Columbus," I said.

"Columbus?" I got worried. "I guess I should have looked at that ticket a little closer. We are headed in the opposite direction. We are going to Chicago. I guess I will need to put you off in Muncie. We will call your parents, and I will see that you get on a bus headed in the right direction. I think one will be along in four or five hours. It should get there before the station closes for the night."

My nine-year-old mind raced. What was I going to do? I cannot tell you the relief I felt when he slowed for a station, picked up the microphone and announced "Franklin." Franklin was the first stop on the way to Columbus. He reached back, smacked me on the knee, and said, "I was just kidding you. We will be in Columbus soon."

I had not been using the bus system long before I discovered that if one took an express bus, time could be shaved off the trip. These particular busses would run non-stop between larger cities unless there was a passenger to disembark in one of the smaller towns on the way. Since I rode this line sort of regularly, I got to know the drivers well. I would sit close to the front and talk with them for at least part of the trip.

There was one occasion when I thought I had been kidnapped by the bus driver. I remember the day like it was yesterday. I was fifteen. This particular time I had received an envelope in the mail which simply contained a bus ticket. Since there was no further instruction from Mom, I assumed she or Dad would meet me at the Greensburg bus station. On this particular Friday, I walked out to the bus when it was announced and handed the driver my ticket as usual, supposing that I was to exit at Greensburg. He smiled and greeted me, tore off and handed me my stub, and welcomed me aboard. I was tired that day so I sat farther back, reclined my seat, and was asleep before we got out of Indianapolis. Somehow I had developed the ability to feel the difference in the road when we neared Greensburg. If I was napping, I would wake up a few minutes before we got to the station, as I did this particular week. I straightened my seat, got my things together, and waited for the bus to stop at the station. When it did not stop, I thought I had misjudged my location, so I sat back to relax. I became alarmed when I heard one of the passengers ask how far we were from Cincinnati. The driver told him that we needed to make a stop in Batesville, and then Cincinnati would be about forty minutes away.

Batesville? I started up from my seat and walked as calmly as I could to the front of the bus. "Did we miss Greensburg?" I asked.

"No," the driver said. "I just decided not to stop. If you want, I can put you off at Batesville. Maybe your parents will pick you up there."

I was in a panic! What other choice did I have? Honestly, I wanted to cry, but fifteen-year-old guys do not cry. I screwed up my courage, sat quietly in my seat, resolved to be off that bus as soon as we stopped. When the door opened, I was off before the driver. Mom was right there to meet me. The driver came off behind me with a huge grin on his face. As it turned out, Mom had worked an elaborate scheme to surprise me with an evening with her and Dad. Since both of them worked at a factory in Batesville, they had decided to have me come to them, and we would have dinner together before going home. She had picked up my ticket at Greensburg and had made arrangements through the agent to get word to the regular driver of her plans. She sent a separate letter to my housemother at the school dorm, asking her to simply hand me the envelope containing the ticket, and not divulge that the ticket was for a different destination. That is the only time I remember having Mom and Dad to myself.

WATCH OUT FOR THAT TRAIN!

One thing that Dale and I enjoyed doing during our early teenage years was to walk into Greensburg on Saturday afternoons. It was about a two-mile walk if we took the usual route. However, if we cut across the golf course and walked the railroad tracks which ran through the middle of the greens, we could cut off about a quarter of a mile. These tracks were a supply line for factories located on the outskirts of town. Trains moved up and down them throughout the week and delivered the goods needed to each. Other than that they were never used.

We had stayed in town later than usual one particular Saturday evening and were hurrying home, so we decided to walk along the tracks to save time. A high trestle bridged the lake in the center of the golf course. Dale and I particularly enjoyed the feeling of danger we got while crossing this trestle. As we stepped onto it, I told Dale that I felt vibrations. "No you don't," he said, looking back. "You know as well as I do that these tracks are not used on the weekends."

We walked on. As we got farther out onto the trestle, I was certain I felt vibrations. I said nothing though, thinking I was just being paranoid for some reason. As we got near to the end of the trestle, a train whistle sounded behind us. We never heard the engine until we heard the whistle. Dale froze and I bolted, dragging him along with me. I was running as fast as I could, hoping I would not miss a cross-tie and fall between them, getting stuck and getting both of us killed.

When I thought we were off the trestle, I jumped, pulling Dale to what I thought would be safety. We barely hit the edge of the lake. We were safe and dry. The train was moving so slowly that the engineer could have stopped in plenty of time. He knew that, but we didn't. As he passed us, he lay on the whistle and waved at us with an ear-to-ear grin. By the way, we took the longer route from that time forward. What was a quarter of a mile anyway? Besides, Mom and Dad had forbidden us to walk on the tracks. They did not find out that we had done so until we were grown.

It was also about this time that I learned to ride a bicycle. Mom had forbidden me to do so, which was exactly what Dale and I needed to challenge me to learn how to ride. Dale had the brand new bike, and I had the determination. We headed for the pavilion at the county fairgrounds across the road from our house. I picked up on the process quickly. As my confidence grew, so did my speed. I flew down the pavilion at breakneck speed.

"Stop!" Dale shouted. I applied the brakes, which did not work. I slammed into a support post, knocking myself out and demolishing Dale's brand new bicycle. I awoke with a knot on my head that could not be hidden from my parents. After discussing it together for a while, Dale informed me that Jane was supposed to pick him up for a week stay in Indianapolis. He suggested that I go in his stead. I agreed.

To cover up our transgressions, Dale placed his wrecked bicycle behind Dad's truck. When Dad ran over it, Dale took the punishment for leaving the bike in his way, and I spent the week (and the next!) recuperating at my sister's house.

ONE UGLY CAR

In my last semester of high school, after we had moved to Florida, Dale acquired an old Ford Falcon. That was one ugly car! It needed a paint job, so Dale painted it orange with a roller. The exhaust was shot and could be heard for a long distance. It had a low rumble that could be felt before it could be heard. Dale was working the night shift at a local egg processing plant. Mom would feel when he had started the car, three miles away, and would have his meal on the table when he got home.

We went everywhere in that car. People knew we were coming. Two events resulted in that car being stamped indelibly in my memory.

I was fascinated with Cindy. She was friendly, cute, and seemed slightly interested in me. I finally asked her out on a double date with Dale and his girlfriend. She agreed to go. The next morning, Dale and I rode to school in his Falcon for the first time. "Are we going in that thing?" Cindy asked. "Yes," I said. She became immediately uninterested and informed me that she would be washing her hair that night and any other night I asked her out. I never got a date with her.

The second incident took place after the graduation party that my aunt and uncle threw for me. I had too good of a time and imbibed too many adult beverages. At two in the morning, I decided I wanted a burger from a local joint. Even though Dale reminded me that the place closed at 11pm, I could not be talked out of going down there so I could see for myself.

Along with being loud and ugly, the car did not have a working gas gauge. Dale had designed a makeshift measuring device, which consisted of a stiff piece of wire with lines on it marking different measurements. Dale would insert this wire into the tank and guess, within a gallon or two, how much was inside. He inserted the wire and informed me that he was on empty. I reminded him that he probably had at least a gallon, and that we should try it. "If we run out of gas, you are pushing," he informed me. Confidently, I agreed.

We went out the dirt road we lived on, down the highway, over the hill and down the other side, and ran out of gas. Since no service stations were open, and since Dale was not about to leave his prized possession alongside the road, I pushed while he steered. I could barely stand up. I simply leaned on the car and made my feet go. I pushed that stupid car two miles up the highway, and down the dirt road as far as my aunt and uncle's house before Dale let me stop.

DRIVING PEOPLE CRAZY

I visited my brother Jerry in Tampa the summer after we moved to Florida. Jerry owned a Honda 305 Superhawk Motorcycle. Growing up, I always wanted to ride a motorcycle, not on the back, but on the front, driving. One hot afternoon, I talked Jerry into letting me ride it with him on the back giving me directions. After he was assured that I knew how to use the brake and the clutch and could change gears, we headed down the street in his development. We got to the end of the street and turned onto a busy boulevard. We proceeded up this street for a couple of blocks, turned into another development, and went to visit one of Jerry's friends. Jerry drove back home. The next morning he was stopped for illegal lights, illegal exhaust, and an illegal helmet. We laughed as we tried to imagine the policeman if he had pulled us over when I was driving. I would probably still be in jail!

Shortly after this incident, when I returned home to Hilliard after a long visit with Jerry, I had another unusual experience. This one was brought on by the fact that a friend and I had again imbibed too many adult beverages. We were watching a Cincinnati Reds' baseball game on television at his father's business, indulging in the beer that Jack had brought with him.

When the game ended and the beer was gone, it was time for Jack to take me home. "Can I drive?" I asked. Without hesitation, Jack agreed. We climbed into his car, he in the passenger seat, and me behind the wheel. He handed me the keys and I started the car. We moved slowly onto the road, Jack giving me verbal instructions.

"Right! Left! Keep it straight! That's it."

As I moved down the road at the breakneck speed of four or five miles per hour, we passed the Federal Aviation Administration Center. The shift had changed, and there were about thirty cars that could not get around me since I was weaving all over the road. As we approached the traffic light at the intersection of the county road we were on and US 1, I somehow got the car onto the grass at the side of the road, and the cars began to pass us. As the first car passed, the driver shouted, "Are you blind?" Jack and I sat there laughing for almost half an hour at my answer, "As a matter of fact..." The next morning Jack phoned me. "Did I let you drive my car last night?" When I told him he had, he simply said, "Man, I'm stupid!"

Another time I drove was while I was attending Toccoa Falls College in northeast Georgia. Bart, one of my friends, owned a big station wagon. One day we came up with a terrific idea that we were sure would astound and amaze the students and faculty of the college. Bart was quite short and could hide on the passenger side of the car. He could peek over the dashboard and see where we were going. He slouched down in the seat, placed one hand on the wheel to guide the car. I sat behind the wheel, both hands on it. I applied the gas and brakes as he instructed, and we drove through the middle of campus right when the last class of the day was letting out. I blew the horn and waved, calling out to people as we went through campus. The street cleared as people realized who was behind the wheel. It was some time before we told anyone how we pulled off that stunt.

A CAR TO REMEMBER

When Ann and I married, she was the proud owner of a 1961 Plymouth Belvedere she had inherited from her grandfather. For those of you who remember the old TV show "Car 54," that was the type of car it was. For those of you who have no idea what I'm talking about, the car was very large, more like a boat, with lots of room inside. "Belvy," as Ann affectionately called her, allowed us to travel many pleasurable miles. Belvy had a few problems, however. For one, the front passenger window would occasionally drop down into the door without notice. The door would have to be taken apart, and the window put back on track. This was particularly inconvenient in Toccoa, Georgia where it rained almost daily. Belvy got about 23 miles to the gallon, and about the same for a quart of oil.

Secondly, the emergency brake was completely shot. There is hardly a level parking place in Toccoa. That model Plymouth had a push button transmission. There was a first, second, drive, and reverse gear. There was also a neutral, but no park. In order to ensure that the car would not roll away when we parked it on a hill, we carried a rock in the trunk. It was our practice for Ann to park the car and place her foot on the brake while

I retrieved the rock from the trunk and placed it in front or behind one of the rear wheels, depending on the direction of the hill. We would then pray that no one would kick the rock out from behind the wheel. When we were ready to leave, we reversed the process. Ann would get into the car, place her foot on the brake again, and I would remove the rock and secure it in the trunk.

Believe it or not, we still miss that car!

CHAPTER 7

MONEY TALKS

Growing up in a large family meant that extra spending money was hard to come by. Mom and Dad usually worked minimum wage jobs, so there was just barely enough to go around for the necessities. We kids seemed to always find creative ways to come up with extra money for luxuries. The girls would babysit, and my older brothers mowed lawns, washed cars, whatever they needed to. Dale and I often collected pop bottles out of the ditches alongside the country roads. We could get two cents apiece for them. Sometimes, however, one would find a slightly shady way to get funds. Creativity ran high in our family as the following three examples of how I got extra money will illustrate.

THE RACKET

My older brother Mike was always fascinated with the gangsters of the 1920's. He often regaled me with tales of how they stole from the rich to make themselves richer. His favorite stories were about the rackets they would contrive to extract funds from people. Perhaps that is where I got the idea to start a racket of my own. It worked pretty well until I got greedy, and then those whom I was extorting blew the whistle on me.

My sister Jane started dating a "nice young man" named Dale. I am not kidding; his name is Dale! She eventually married him. I don't know if his name motivated me to take advantage of him in order to get back at someone else named Dale, or if I just saw an opportunity. At any rate, as they got "chummy," I got an idea. With so many kids around, privacy of any kind was at a premium. My older brothers did not bother Jane and Dale much, but little brother Dale and I could be real pains! I knew that if I left the room, Dale would, too. So I came up with an idea that I hoped would work, and it did. When Jane and Dale would sit cozily on the couch, I would wedge myself between them and begin to talk incessantly. I also insisted that Dale play with me rather than pay attention to Jane. A few minutes of this kind of behavior, and Dale would come up with a quarter. Upon receiving it, I would smile and politely excuse myself, and brother Dale would follow. I saw to it that he got a nickel from my spoils.

Things went along quite well for a couple of months, and then it happened. I got greedy. It was near Christmas time, and I wanted some extra money to buy myself something nice. Dale showed up and sat on the couch beside Jane. I wedged myself between them, and the ritual began. When Dale produced the quarter, I politely informed him that the price for my absence just went up to a dollar. Jane simply got up, walked into the kitchen, and informed Mom of my extortion tactics. It was not a dollar that I got that day!

THE SAFE WAY

Mike was always kind of greedy. He hoarded anything, especially money. When he got a job at Sears, he purchased a little tin safe with a combination lock on the door. He felt that Dale and I needed to be kept out of his stash. He selected a combination that he was certain we could not figure out and challenged us to do so.

"If you can open this safe," he said, "you can have any amount of money you want." Of course, we knew that he meant that if we could open the safe that particular day. He did not say that, however. Dale and I worked on that safe for weeks until we finally figured out the combination. Rather than getting greedy and getting caught, we decided to extract only a little money at a time. Mike drank quite heavily, and we knew that if we were careful he would never know that he was being robbed blind. He would think he got into his stash without remembering. If we wanted a soft drink, a candy bar, or an afternoon at the skating rink or movie theater, we "borrowed" from Mike's safe. He never caught on.

MOVIE LOGIC

Greensburg, Indiana boasted one movie theater. It was a small one right downtown on the square. If everybody inhaled and did not exhale, the Tree Theater might have held fifty people. Saturday morning matinees were the thing to do. Since money was tight, I came up with a plan to make our meager funds go farther.

It did not take long for me to recognize that the girl that worked behind the combination ticket and concession counter was fascinated with the little blind boy. The fact that she was incredibly gullible was no small matter. As Dale and I stood in front of her, taking our turn at the ticket window, the idea hit me.

"You know," I said, "I think I should be allowed to get in for half price since I am only going to listen to the movie and not watch it." She agreed with my logic and sold me my ticket for half price. I got in that way for several weeks until one fateful Saturday when I sashayed up to the window, purchased my ticket from her, and the manager, who happened to be the owner, saw what was happening. No matter how much she and I explained our logic, he did not buy it. In fact, I could not get into another movie until I paid back all of those previous admissions I had cheated him out of. Busted again!

CHAPTER 8

BOY, COULD MY MOM COOK!

Mom was really a good cook! I still remember the smell of her homemade bread. When we lived near other people, it seemed that the scent of fresh bread filled the entire neighborhood. Kids and adults alike would just happen to be nearby when the bread came out of the oven.

Mom's pie crusts would melt in your mouth. I can still almost taste her rhubarb pie, out of the oven long enough to cool where it could be cut. A big piece of that pie and a tall glass of cold milk, and I was in heaven!

While Mom was a great cook, she did make some mistakes that will go down in Thompson family history.

SOME POWERFUL SPAGHETTI

We had just moved again! The place where we lived was quite rural. The county was sparsely populated, and the high school Jane would be attending was several miles away. It was the custom of this particular county that when a new student moved into the area, the School Board would dispatch a Trustee out to the home to meet him or her, fill out the necessary paperwork, and welcome the student to the school. That is just what happened one particular evening.

We did not have cooking gas or electricity in the house yet since we had just moved in. Mom often waited several weeks before installing these conveniences. It was a cold winter evening, so the wood stove in the living room was burning steadily, warming every crevice of that room to a toasty, drowsy comfort.

Thinking the Trustee would not take long, Mom placed a large unopened can of spaghetti on top of the heating stove to warm just before he arrived. It would be our supper when he left. It turned out that the Trustee was a slow, methodical, older man. As he took his time, Mike watched the sealed can swell as the heat built up inside. Everyone else in the room was focusing on Jane and the Trustee.

When the can exploded and whizzed past the Trustee's ear, he jumped, dropping the huge pile of papers on the floor. Spaghetti flew everywhere, miraculously not hitting anyone. The walls, floor, and ceiling of the living room were covered with a red mess. When Mom determined that no one was hurt, she laughed uncontrollably. We all joined in, even the Trustee. I do not remember what we had for supper that night, but I do remember Mom still scraping spaghetti off the walls and ceiling when we moved out of that house. She was never quite sure she found it all.

THE SECRET IS IN THE FILLING

We all loved Mom's pancakes! Each one was as big as a dinner plate! One was all we needed. One particular day we begged her to make some of her wonderful pancakes for us. She finally agreed and got out her ingredients, including the powdered milk.

Things were tough for us, so we received commodity groceries. We got twenty-five pounds of flour, a huge can of peanut butter, several cans of something they called meat, butter, cheese, rice, oats, and a huge box of powdered milk.

Mom mixed the ingredients and began to cook those wonderful pancakes. We could not get enough of them! I am not sure how many I had eaten when Mom snatched all of the plates off the table and threw the contents away with a flourish. We were puzzled. She did not want to tell us what the problem was. "I think you have had enough," was all she would say.

After some more loud protests, she showed my brothers the problem. As she pointed to the open box of powdered milk, they all ran for the outhouse to throw up. Mice had gotten into the box and left their droppings. Those pancakes had a special secret filling. It was years before I could eat another pancake!

BREAD THAT WILL STICK TO YOUR RIBS

As I said at the beginning of this chapter, Mom could make some delicious bread. Most of the time, anyway. One weekend, I invited some friends to come home with me from the school for the blind. Mom knew how much they loved her homemade bread, so she whipped up a nice loaf. I am not sure what went wrong. That loaf of bread was as hard as a rock and just as heavy. One of my friends, Phil, ate a piece "just to be polite." The rest of us politely declined. Mom threw the rest of the loaf out into the back yard for the neighborhood dogs. They would not even eat it! Phil was not very hungry for the rest of the weekend.

CHAPTER 9

ANIMAL STORIES

  About the same time I got in trouble for all of those rusty tools, Mom and Dad took in a boarder. The girls had moved out for a few months, so he got their room. I do not remember much about the guy, but I definitely remember his dog. It was a little shaggy mutt named Spot. He was a gentle dog. We could play with him, pull his ears and tail, you get the picture. The only quirk this little dog had was that if anyone under five feet tall walked out into the yard with anything that looked edible, he would summarily bite that person on the left leg, and while his victim grabbed for that leg, Spot would grab and eat whatever was in that person's hand. I am not sure why we kids could not get the idea through our heads that Spot was going to bite us if we went into the yard with food. After several biting incidents, Dale announced that the next time Spot bit him he was going to bite him back.

  Dale was a calculating sort. He actually began plotting a way to get Spot to bite him. The very next day after his announcement, he walked into the back yard carrying a large handful of crackers. He had hardly gotten off the back steps when I heard a loud yell from Dale, followed by a loud yelp from the dog, and then the sound of Dale spitting. He had done as he promised. He had bitten Spot on the back of the head, leaving quite a large bald spot. Spot never bit us again.

FOR THE BIRDS

I must confess that as a small child I was afraid of chickens, a fear that I mistakenly confided to Dale one day in a moment of weakness. Dale said he would help me get over my fear. I actually trusted him!

A couple of days later we were playing in the back yard. I had forgotten all about the chickens since Mom kept them shut up in a chicken house most of the time. What had prompted me to tell Dale about my fear was the fact that one of the roosters had gotten out. As we played, Dale wandered closer and closer to the chicken house. I heard them but thought nothing about it. After all, Mom had prohibited us from going into that building. I reasoned that Dale would never break one of Mom's rules. Dale eased over to the door and opened it slightly. "Come here, Sammy," he said innocently.

Like a fool, I walked over to him. He pushed me inside and closed the door. He quickly ran inside to tell Mom that I had gone into the chicken house. Meanwhile, I was paralyzed with fear. Chickens were all around me! Thousands of them! Actually, there were probably less than a hundred, but to me there were thousands. They fluttered, they squawked, they even bumped into me. And then I heard it. A sound I had never heard before. It came from a corner of the building opposite me. What I heard was a loud monster with a voice like a foghorn. I thought that whatever it was would surely eat me. This "monster" was actually a new goose that Mom had acquired.

Fear or not, I decided I had to get out of there before that monster got so hungry that it ate me and all of those horrible chickens. I threw the door open and bolted for the house. The problem was that I did not quite know where the house was since I was not supposed to be in that part of the yard. When I threw the door open and ran, the chickens and goose surged out behind me. It was quite a picture: a little frightened blind boy running across the yard, bumping into trees, the side of the outhouse, the tool shed, with fowl right on his heels. I finally fell into the creek, which brought the fowl up short.

Mom rounded up the chickens and goose, and then rounded me up. Somehow Dale convinced her that he was nowhere near that chicken house and that he had seen me go in all by myself. I vowed to get even, and get even I did. However, it was totally by accident.

HERE KITTY, KITTY!

Mom regularly fed a panther in our back yard. She didn't know it was a panther at first. She had a habit of taking the table scraps out beside the shed after each meal and dumping them on the ground for all of the wild animals to enjoy after dark.

Late in the afternoon one spring day, she looked out the kitchen window to see a young, beautiful kitten helping itself to the scraps. Mom was always a softy when it came to cats, a tendency that I definitely did not inherit. After that day, she would pour out the scraps and call, "Here Kitty, Kitty!" She would then retreat inside, and the "kitty" would help itself.

Over a period of weeks the kitty would be standing at the edge of the woods behind the shed when Mom would pour out the scraps. It would never come into the yard until Mom went back into the house.

As spring turned into summer, Kitty got bigger and her markings became more defined. Mom had been feeding a panther! Wisely, she continued to do so, figuring that it was better for the cat to eat table scraps than one of us kids. She later told me that there were times when she considered stopping the free meals and sending us out into the woods to play after the animal had had a few days of fasting.

Kitty had it made, so she took up residence on our property. Each morning in the fall, when my older brothers and sisters headed up the hill in the early morning darkness to catch the school bus, they would often spy two bright eyes staring at them from a tree line on one side or other of the path. As we played in the woods, she often briefly appeared, darting through a clearing, or we would spot her behind or in a tree. We even got used to her screams in the night. Most of us, anyway. Dale was terrified. If the truth were to be known, so was I, but that was information I decided Dale would never be privy to. Or would he?

One afternoon Dale and I were playing "horsey" with some old ball bats of our brothers in the long lane which led up to the bridge at the base of the hill we had to climb to exit The Hollow. Since we were not permitted beyond the bridge without supervision, we had turned around on our horseys and headed back toward the house when it happened. The scream came loud and clear, piercing through the woods, echoing off the trees, exaggerated by the vast number of them. It was reinforced by the human screams of my brothers who were playing in the woods farther up the hill. My brothers had been playing in a certain spot in the woods where the panther hung out and had somehow surprised her. She screamed and held her ground. They screamed and ran. So did Dale and I! Let me tell you, this little blind kid could run! The last thing I remember, until I got into the house, was Dale begging me to slow down so that I could get eaten with him. "Don't let him eat me by myself," he called. I had gone inside and gotten a drink of water before Dale arrived to complain to Mom that I wouldn't wait for him.

Shortly after this incident, we moved, and the panther started foraging the nearby farms for food. It wasn't long before the local paper reported that a large panther had been shot while trying to steal an animal from one of the neighboring farms. Kitty was no more.

SNAKE!

The last time we moved into The Hollow, the house had been unoccupied for quite some time. Teenagers would venture down to the house for all kinds of mischief, but mostly, since the doors had no locks on them, and the teenagers left them open when they left, animals pretty much ran the place. It was no surprise that there was a lot of cleaning up that needed to take place before we could move back into the house. Mom thought she had done a pretty good job of ridding the house of all the varmints before the furniture was actually put into place. The only ones she was certain were still there were the bees in the hive located inside the living room wall. We would just have to put up with them until one of us got tired of the other.

About a week after we moved in, Mom and Dad headed off to work in Columbus, leaving Bill in charge of us younger kids. I remember the things that happened next like it was yesterday. I had been outside playing and had just entered the front door, which had been left open since it was a warm summer day. We had no screen door, which was a real blessing on this occasion. Bill was sitting in an old wooden rocking chair directly across the living room from the open front door. He was chatting absent-mindedly with Dan, Mike, and Jerry about something insignificant when he looked down at the floor. "Snake!" he screamed at the top of his lungs, and jumped straight into the air from a seated position. The adrenalin must have been rushing. He leapt across the room, clearing my head and landing outside the front door on his feet. My other brothers thought that there was something wrong with him until they looked where he was excitedly and speechlessly pointing. Wrapped around the front leg of the chair was a huge copperhead poised to strike. That snake was killed instantly.

When Mom was shown the snake that evening, she said, "That explains the snake skin I found in the corner of the living room!"

"HEY MOM, WHAT'S FOR SUPPER?"

There were always animals around the property. Animals for eating, that is. Mom and Dad told us that it was all right to get attached to the livestock as long as we realized that we would eventually need to help catch our pets so that we could eat them. One goat that I had as a pet, which we did eventually eat, was a nanny goat, appropriately named Nanny. Mom would stake her out under the oak tree beside the creek where she could eat grass and get water to drink. This also kept her from wandering off into the woods and possibly getting eaten by some predator. I would walk out to pet Nanny, and she would walk around and around me, causing her chain to wind around my legs. I do not know why I did not learn that she would do this, but I never did. I would be trapped until one of my siblings decided to release me, or Mom came out to do so. I spent quite a bit of time "tied up" with Nanny.

I think goats were Mom's favorite animals to raise and cook. We ate a lot of goat when I was growing up. One particular goat, a billy, appropriately named Billy, was a thorn in Mom's side. She was very pregnant with my brother Dale when Dad brought him home. He had gotten him in some kind of deal while trading for a car, I think. This particular goat had a habit of butting anybody who got in his way. For some reason this goat was allowed to roam free in the yard. However, every time Mom went out the back door to the outhouse, Billy would butt her into the creek. After a week or two of this treatment, she informed Dad that the next time that happened she was going to single-handedly kill, butcher, and cook that goat for supper. Dad laughed. The next evening we were eating goat steak.

Shopping for the family was quite easy for Mom. Just how easy it was became apparent to me when I was about three. I was sitting in the kitchen with Mom, chattering away as toddlers do when I asked, "Hey Mom, what's for supper?" She walked to the back door, opened it, looked out into the back yard, and announced "Duck." We ate duck that evening.

IN A PIG'S EYE!

Dad found a pig. You read it right, Dad found a pig. While driving home one Saturday afternoon, Dad spotted a half-grown pig walking along the road. Concerned about its safety, he stopped to survey the situation. There were no homes in the immediate vicinity. Dad pondered what to do. On impulse, he opened the trunk of the car. The pig stood there and watched him, making no attempt to run off. Dad walked over, scratched its back and walked slowly toward the car. The pig followed, Dad's hand lightly on its back. It was obvious that this was someone's pet. The pig actually helped Dad get it into the trunk! Dad checked with farmers within a ten-mile radius of where he found the pig, and he belonged to none of them. Dad brought him home and named him Pork.

Since we had no pigs at the time, we had no pen for Pork. Dad let him wander around the yard, intending to build a pen for him, which he never got around to doing. Pork was quite clean, confining his wallowing and other business to one corner of the yard. Like a dog, he greeted Dad every time he came into the back yard. Dad would talk to him, pet him, and scratch his back. If we had company, Pork would pull on Dad's pants leg until Dad excused himself from visiting and gave him some attention.

Pork had one problem. He was a kleptomaniac. He picked up whatever was lying on the ground and hide it. We all learned not to leave anything in the yard that he could pick up, or we might never find it again. Pork particularly loved Dad's tools, especially his wrenches. Maybe it was because they were shiny. Dad kept his tools in pristine condition.

Dad was always working on some old car. He would slide under the car, placing the tools he would need on the ground beside him. He would be concentrating on his work to the point that he did not see Pork wandering up to the work site. He only noticed after a particular wrench he needed was missing. He would interrupt his work to look for the missing tool. He usually found them and promised Pork that he would enjoy the bacon he was going to eat.

We kept Pork for quite some time. While Mom and Dad had always said that it was all right to have farm animals as pets, we went quite some time without meat because of Dad's attachment to that pig.

THE ABC'S OF BEES

I was not always very bright. There was a beautiful patch of clover in the front yard where I would sit for hours listening to the honeybees gathering nectar. The problem was that I not only listened to them, but I also tried to pick them up to see what they felt like when they lighted on the clover flowers beside me (remember,

I was a curious child). Every time I got stung between my thumb and index finger on my left hand. I would go crying to Mom and she would fix me up. At least that is the way things went for a while, until she discovered that I was deliberately picking up the bees.

"If you pick up another bee," she told me, "I will have to spank you." I remember very well the last bee I would ever pick up.

RIDE 'EM, COWGIRL!

When I was about eight years old, our cousins from Florida came to visit. Six-year-old Darleen decided she wanted to hang around Dale and me. Of course, at that age, girls were a real annoyance. We tried everything we could to discourage her from hanging around with us, from beating her up to leaving her in the woods when we played. Nothing worked.

Dad's sister, Aunt Dorothy, had purchased a bull calf, which Mom and Dad had graciously permitted her to keep in a small pasture out behind our house. Star was a friendly sort. Aunt Dorothy had purchased him when he was a few days old, and Mom had raised him. We castrated him when he was old enough, and he grew like crazy. He was a gentle giant. He must have thought he was a dog. If we were in the pasture, he followed us around wanting to be petted.

One particular day, we were playing in the pasture, and Star came over for some attention. As I was petting him, Darleen asked, "Can you ride him?" "Sure," I lied. "I ride him all the time!" Star had never been ridden. I knew that he would stand calmly while she mounted him because we climbed on him all the time. I was not sure what would happen after that.

He stood very still while she climbed on his back. She sat atop this huge creature and asked, "How do I make him go?" "Kick him in the sides," I told her. Darleen did everything with a flourish. She stuck each leg out as far as she could and brought them together with as much force as possible. Star jumped straight up into the air. Darleen went sailing over his head and landed several feet in front of him, right smack in the middle of one of his deposits. Star bent his head down, grabbed a mouthful of grass, and looked at her with wonder. Darleen was not hurt, but her pride was. She ran crying to her mother and, no matter how hard we tried, would not play with us anymore.

TO THE DOGS

I have used two dog guides in my lifetime. This section will give some insight into a few of the things you will seldom hear about these special animals.

Muffin, The Wonder Dog
I received Muffin just before I headed off to college in northeast Georgia. She was quite the con artist! She learned shortly after I brought her home that some people would react if she acted hurt when I corrected her. Correction is administered by the application of a quick jerk on the leash, which briefly tightens the slip collar. Properly administered, it does not hurt the dog. Muffin would lie down, gag, and quiver after the most minor act of discipline. Mom especially reacted when I found it necessary to correct Muffin, until the day she betrayed herself by over acting a little too much.

I had arrived at Toccoa Falls College a few days early in order to get oriented to the campus and get Muffin settled in. Doreen, my girlfriend at the time, was there also, and I was interested in spending some time with her before school started. As Mom, Dad, Doreen,

Muffin, and I toured the campus, Muffin spotted a cat at the top of a flight of stairs. She did what dogs do naturally. She tried to chase the cat. She attempted to dash up the stairs with me holding the harness. I stopped her and made her sit on the third step up. This was a major infraction, so I dropped her harness handle, grabbed the leash with both hands, and planted my feet for a serious correction. Doreen begged me not to hurt the "cute little puppy." Muffin had things timed perfectly for her little act. She knew how long it took me to get her to sit, to position myself, and to apply the discipline. This particular day, however, I was delayed by the necessity of explaining why I had to correct this cute little puppy. When Muffin had waited the normal length of time, she fell backward off the steps, rolled onto her back, and began to gag and quiver. I had not touched her! She was quite the actress. Doreen began laughing hysterically, exclaiming, "That dog is more of a ham than you!"

A few days later, I was summoned to the financial office to sign some papers. It was raining cats and dogs, pardon the pun. I waited for the rain to slack off, and then Muffin and I headed for the administration building. I signed the necessary papers, and we headed back to the dorm. I stood under the awning outside of the building, waiting for the rain to slow down again. When the time came I said, "Muffin, forward."

Muffin stepped out beautifully and then spied a squirrel. About that same time, the rain began to come down in buckets. Muffin lit out after that squirrel like a shot out of a cannon with me in tow. I was holding onto the harness with my left hand, leaning forward to retrieve the leash that I had dropped, while running to keep up with Muffin. I could not slow her down! We ran through parts of the campus I knew nothing about, until Muffin lost the squirrel. We were lost, and I was very angry! As

I tried to get my bearings, a little old lady came out of one of the houses we were near and informed me that we were on a hill way up above the center of campus. She offered her umbrella and we started down the hill. I would not let Muffin under the umbrella. I figured she deserved to be wet!

Muffin did not last long. After the flood on the campus at Toccoa Falls College in November of 1977, she had to be returned to the school from which she came.

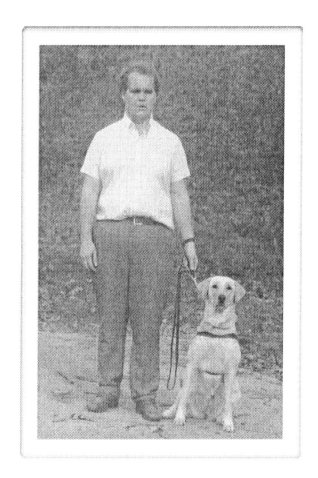

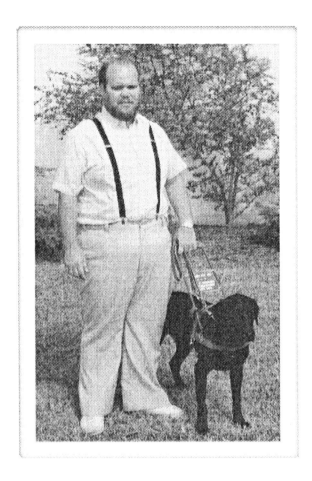

All in Good Stride

I received my second dog, Strider, in 1988. What a dog he was! We were together for ten years and I could not have asked for a better guide. He seemed able to anticipate my desire and fulfill it without me having to say much. There were a couple of times, however, when I think I might have shot him if I had had a gun (just kidding!).

The first incident occurred upon his first follow-up evaluation after coming home with me. His trainer met us at my office, and we headed out for a little walk. I was dressed up since I would not be going home before catching a plane as I headed to my first-ever meeting as a member of the National Advisory Committee on

Disabilities Ministries at the national office of The Christian and Ministry Alliance in Nyack, New York. Strider was excited to see his trainer again. He was having trouble focusing on his task. I finally got him settled down, and we started through our route, one that we had practiced many times. I wanted him to look great for his trainer. We were doing quite well until Strider stopped in the middle of a block. He would not move! I did all of the proper things: I checked with my feet to determine if there was a curb or drop off, I checked overhead to see if there was a clearance problem, I listened for the possibility of traffic crossing in front of us, and then I checked out the dog. All was clear. As I gave the forward command, I felt a warm sensation in my left shoe. Strider's aim was perfect! He filled my shoe with a warm, yellow, smelly liquid. I had no time to go home and shower before leaving for the airport. Needless to say, the seat next to me on the plane stayed empty.

A couple of years later, Ann and I were traveling representing Clearer Vision Ministries, Inc. We had stopped at a hotel for the night. I had just gotten settled into bed when Strider began to nudge me like he needed to go outside. Since I had taken him out a few minutes earlier, I did not hurry. The sound I soon heard brought me to my feet. I told Ann that I would clean up the mess when I got back inside, but I felt I should get the dog outside, let him finish up, and correct him first. I slipped my foot into my house slipper, which I had left by the exit door. It felt warm and wet! Strider got nothing on the carpet, but my new slipper was ruined!

During this time, Ann and I were involved in singles ministry at the church we were attending. They all loved Strider, too, and were faithful to get him something for Christmas. One year, a couple of the young ladies went together and purchased the largest rawhide chew bone I have ever seen. They presented it to him at our annual Christmas party. We all thought that it would last for months. Wrong! He consumed that entire bone in one evening. This was a Saturday night.

Ann was playing the piano for the church's Christmas musical that year and I was singing. As the choir prayed together before going into the sanctuary, a pungent, unmistakable odor wafted through the crowded room. That chew bone had given Strider the worst case of gas I ever remember any dog having! I thought that he must have expelled all of the gas he had, and would ever have, in his system, and we should be all right from that point on. Wrong!

The choir assembled, each in his or her proper place in the choir loft. My place was in the bass section on the back row, the section that backed up to the wall separating the choir loft from the baptistry. Strider lay obediently under the pew. As we sat for part of the narration, I noticed a faint smell coming from under the pew. It grew to an almost "eye watering" intensity and filtered throughout the entire choir loft. Some of the women gagged slightly and some of the men, including me, choked back laughter.

As if that were not bad enough, Strider got an itch during one of the most poignant parts of the narration. As he scratched that itch, his harness began to thump the wooden wall behind him. As it got louder and louder, the choir director got more and more angry. I tried to reach Strider, but he had curled up way under the pew. I finally reached him and pulled him out away from the wall. Thanks to Strider, and much to my relief, I was never recruited to sing in that choir again.

You can't tell me dogs have short memories! Every Christmas, we would get Strider a little something. It was not for his benefit, just some pretend sentiment that Ann and I would go through to make our day a little novel. We would give him our gift, usually a chew bone, and he would lie in a corner happily gnawing it to bits while we opened our gifts. This same year we did not get him anything because of the large bone the girls had given him. We did not think it would really matter.

We opened our gifts as usual. This time Strider was constantly sticking his face into our packages to see what was in them. We could not get him to go away. When the space under the tree was empty, Strider gave a verbal huff and looked at me with disgust. He went into our bedroom, lay down on his bed, and pouted. He really pouted! When I went in to check on him and tried to pet him, he moved away. I was not very popular for a couple of days. He would work for me, but when I removed his harness, he would go off and sulk. He got something for Christmas every year after that.

Strider gave me much joy and freedom before it was necessary for him to retire in 1999. Because of him, I was able to enjoy events and activities that had previously not been possible. I still miss him.

****

The next few chapters of this book are not especially funny, but they are necessary. They will show you why I can laugh now. I trust you will emerge from the following pages with a new understanding of what Christ can do in and with a life when that life is turned over to Him.

CHAPTER 10

SCHOOL DAYS

THE DAY I REALIZED I WAS "DIFFERENT"

    Summer days in The Hollow were usually wonderful! We boys would spend long hours playing in the woods or in the front yard. As we went up the lane towards the bridge that crossed the creek, there was a large field off to the right that Mom used as a garden at times. When Mom was not using it as a garden, we used that field for baseball and any other activity our imaginations could conjure up.

    One summer day when I was five, my brothers grabbed their ball, bat, and gloves, and headed out the front door to play baseball. I followed them as I always did. I would be given a glove and sent out into right field. I stood there for as long as they played, thinking I was making a contribution to the game. I actually did catch a ball one day, totally by accident. One of my brothers hit a line drive that flew right at me and dropped into my extended glove. Instinctively, I closed my hand around it. My brothers and I could not believe it!

    This particular morning I went out the door behind my brother Mike. He stopped at the bottom of the steps, looked at me, and said, "You can't play baseball!" "Why not?" I asked. "Because you can't see the ball," he replied. I was surprised by this statement, and shattered by the fact that I was not going to be allowed to play with my brothers. This was the first time I recall being singled out as different. It was a confusing and lonely feeling.

I walked into the house with tears in my eyes and headed to the kitchen where Mom was peeling potatoes. I remember standing behind her trying to control my emotions. "Does Jesus love me?" I asked her.

My family was a religious family, but we did not know Christ personally. At the end of the day, we would all be summoned to the living room where Mom read us a chapter from a fictional novel and then a chapter from an old children's Bible storybook. We would then kneel in front of the chairs and couch, and all of us would pray aloud at the same time. We went to church on Sundays, but I do not recall ever hearing of the need for a personal relationship with Christ until I was in the sixth grade. I was taught that if I were good I would go to Heaven; if I was not, then I would go to Hell. I heard the stories about Jesus healing blind men and wondered what bad thing I had done that he would not heal me. Now I was feeling unloved and rejected by my brothers. When I walked into that kitchen, my five-year-old mind was trying to sort out some very difficult thoughts.

Mom put down her knife, turned to face me, picked me up and hugged me. "Of course He loves you!" "Then why did He make me blind?" Mom just held me and cried. She did not have an answer for me. I would spend years trying to find the answer to that question.

OFF TO SCHOOL

I could not wait to start school! Each day that my brothers and sisters trudged out of the house early in the morning, I wished I was with them. I wanted to take my lunch box with its cold bacon sandwich up that hill and wait for the bus. I wanted to sit in a desk and learn new and mysterious things. I wanted to ride the big bus home every day.

When my parents told me that I was a "big boy" and would be starting school, I was ecstatic! I was finally going to get to do all of those things I had looked forward to. And then it happened. I was informed that I would not be riding the big bus. I would not be carrying my lunch. I would not be coming home every evening. I would be going away to a residential school in Indianapolis, about 60 miles away. The only thing I would get to do that I had looked forward to was sit in a desk and learn mysterious things. Nevertheless, in spite of all of the disappointment, I looked forward to starting school.

For some reason I cannot recall, I started my first year of school at the Indiana School for the Blind two weeks late. I sat in the back seat of the car doing everything I could to keep from jumping out of my skin. I am sure that those sixty miles were the longest miles of my parents' lives. "Are we almost there?" "Can you speed up, Daddy?" "Why don't you just run the stop light?"

We finally arrived! I didn't even hug my parents goodbye! I turned and waved and said something to them as I was escorted up the stairs to my classroom. I was finally there! I was introduced to my teacher, Mrs. Wyatt, and my classmates. The students were working on their alphabet when I entered the room. Since I was two weeks late and had no clue what I was supposed to be doing, Mrs. Wyatt showed me my seat and gave me a bar of modeling clay to play with. "Do something with this," she said.

Sitting in front of me was a girl with beautiful, long blond hair. I had observed my older brothers and the way they treated my sisters. I had also listened attentively to many conversations between them, and knew that the reason girls existed was to make it possible for boys to be mischievous without having to always pick on each other. I touched Elaine's hair and the clay on my desktop that I had formed into a ball. And then the idea occurred to me. I simply grabbed the ball of clay in my right hand and a big handful of her hair in my left. I started at the end of her hair, wrapped it securely around the ball of clay, pressed it into place, and began rolling it altogether, quickly reaching her head. Elaine screamed, and Mrs. Wyatt rushed to see what I had done. She quickly removed me from the room, took me down the hall, and introduced me to our principal, who introduced me to "The Board of Education." I had been in school a whole five minutes! Later that day during recess, I asked Elaine if she would be my girlfriend. She said she would.

NEW LIVING ARRANGEMENTS

After class was over that first day, I was shown my dormitory room. I would be sharing a dorm with about twenty other blind boys, and a room with two of them. I was used to being the only blind person moving around a room. Needless to say, it was a challenge when all of us tried to get somewhere at the same time. I felt like a pinball in a machine! I also learned that I lacked some social skills. Between the time I got to the dorm after school and bedtime, I was spanked for breaking one boy's toy, for throwing a wooden block through a window, and for talking to my two roommates after lights out. It was not a good first day at school!

'TIS THE SEASON TO BE NAUGHTY

My "relationship" with Elaine lasted until I met Leigh. I remember when and how it happened. Leigh and I were paired up to walk down the aisle of the auditorium together for the Christmas program. As we sat together during rehearsal, I asked her if she would be my girlfriend. She said she would. I asked her if she would like to come home with me and sleep in my attic. She said she would ask her mommy. Her mommy said no. In spite of that rejection, our love lasted through the Christmas program.

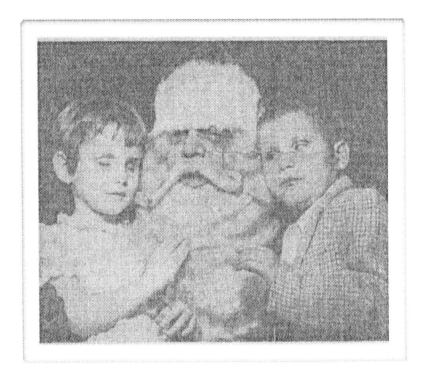

It was during this Christmas season that I revealed Santa's true identity. Despite the fact that I had broken her heart, Elaine was still willing to sit on Santa's lap with me. As I waited in line for my turn, I kept thinking there was something familiar about Santa's voice. As Elaine and I sat on his lap I reached up to touch his beard, and then it hit me. "You're not Santa!" I exclaimed. I pulled his beard, which came away from his face. "You are the janitor!" He was the janitor! Needless to say, I did not get a candy cane that day.

HOW OLD ARE YOU?

My third grade teacher, Miss Carson, was a fantastic teacher! The problem was that I thought she was so old! One day I asked her, "How old are you?" "I'm thirty one," she told me. "Wow! You're old!"

I took my wife by the school to visit years later when I was thirty-one. We ran into Miss Carson. "How old are you?" she asked me. "Thirty one," I said. Then I remembered. I knew what was coming next. "Wow! You're old!" Suddenly thirty-one did not seem so old after all.

While Miss Carson was a great teacher, she had no appreciation for the songs and jokes that my dad and brothers taught me on my rare trips home for the weekend. Whenever I shared one of them during "Show and Tell" time, I would be sent down to have another conversation with "The Board of Education." It got to the point that I was not permitted to share with the class until I had shared with her privately first. Later, when I was in high school, Miss Carson was my English Composition teacher. It is she that I credit for teaching me to think and express myself in vivid imagery. She drilled into her students that we lived in a "sighted world," and we needed to be able to communicate in a way that was acceptable in that world.

"PLAY IT AGAIN, SAM!"

When I was in the fourth grade, my Aunt Dorothy gave me a clarinet that belonged to one of my cousins who had become uninterested in it. This sparked a love affair with music that has lasted a lifetime. It also was the gateway for me to join the school band. When I began taking band classes in the fourth grade, Doc Appleton (his real name) was the teacher. Doc was an older man, probably in his 70's, when I began taking music classes from him. I don't know anyone who didn't love Doc! He was a firm, but loving teacher, a perfectionist who expected the best effort out of anyone he was teaching. He had a knack for knowing if one was not really trying. The result was an excellent concert band and a smaller jazz combo, both award winning.

TEENAGE YEARS

My life between the ages of 12 and 21 was turbulent, to put it mildly. This turbulence will be explained in the following chapter. There were some incredibly funny things that happened during this time, however, that, now that I am past them, make me laugh just to think of them.

By the time I got to seventh grade, Doc had retired and the process of rapidly changing band directors began. During my eighth grade year, we had a director who decided that a concert band was not enough. What the Indiana School for the Blind needed was a marching band! It has been proven that it is possible to have a marching band made up of blind and visually impaired students, but it takes creativity, ingenuity, and some real thinking outside the box. Mr. Barnstorm, who had obviously not taught blind students before, plunged ahead, apparently lacking all of these qualities.

His first attempt was to put the percussion section in front, the theory being that we all could follow the sound, march in a straight line, and play pretty. The problem? Three of the four drummers were totally blind. The result? Each one of us marched to a different drummer.

The next solution was to tie our wrists together with a sighted guide at the end of each line. The problem? Not only is it difficult for drummers to drum with their wrists tied to the person next to them, it is difficult for a trumpet player to play while tied to a slide trombone player. The result? Chaos, confusion, and some amazing displays of contortion.

Mr. Barnstorm was not about to give up! He had one more plan he was sure would work. He had the carpentry shop provide him with long pieces of dowel rod. He secured student volunteers who were not a part of the band to assist. These guys had one simple task to perform: one would hold each end of a dowel rod while the band would stand in formation, bellies pressed firmly against the rod and march. The problem was two-fold. It had rained the night before this fateful practice, and there were large puddles on each side of the road we were to march down, and the cheerleaders were practicing not far from where we were. The result? We all marched along pretty well for about fifty yards until the fellows who were guiding us caught a glimpse of the cheerleaders practicing. Their distraction resulted in the entire band marching through a large puddle, kicking up muddy water and having a blast! No matter how loudly Mr. Barnstorm blew his ever present whistle, we were determined to finish the number we were playing, and finish we did. The idea of a marching band was also finished after that attempt.

WELCOME TO THE "DORM"ICILE

Being a bored teenager is always a challenge. Being a bored teenager at a school for the blind over the weekend when most of your friends have gone home is another story. It was during these times when those of us who remained on the campus got into mischief. There is one particular Sunday I will never forget. It was a cool fall afternoon. We got tired of watching football on TV and decided to go out and play it instead. There weren't enough of us to make up two teams, so we divided as evenly as possible. Half of us took off our shirts and the other half left them on. That way we could tell the teams apart. The very first play, we lost the ball. We just tackled each other, hoping someone had it. While we were in a dog pile, one of the guys found the ball and started running, his head down, toward the "goal" which was the metal post holding up a basketball hoop. He found it, head first. When we got him up, finally, we found the ball, and realized we were all pretty beaten up. The housemother sent us all to the infirmary to get patched up. We were told we were never to play football again without proper supervision.

Those cold winter days and evenings when it was just too nasty to go outside also contributed to boredom. That was when creative juices would flow and mischief reigned supreme! If you are reading this as one who thinks that blind kids cannot get into mischief, you are in for a huge awakening! One of the most puzzling things that ever happened to me caused me, and my housefather, to think I had lost my mind.

Our bedrooms were sparsely furnished. There were two metal beds, two dressers, and two chairs. Lockers were built into the wall to store clothing. One cold December evening, I had actually been studying for several hours. I don't know what had come over me! I went up to my room, ready to take a shower and fall into bed early. When I got into my room, I could not find my bed! Knowing something was up, I started going around the room, carefully feeling my way, expecting what, I didn't really know. I found my bed! The dressers had been moved against the wall, placed just far enough apart for my bed to be set on top of them. I smiled to myself, figuring someone was getting even with me for something I had done. I casually went downstairs and asked the housefather, who had a sense of humor, to help me lift down the bed. He came upstairs with me, and we found the room as it was supposed to be. He laughed and went back to watch the rest of his TV program. I left with him, explaining that the bed had been on top of the dressers. I was not out of the room more than a couple of minutes. When I returned, the bed was back on top of the dressers. I marched back down the stairs for the housefather, who returned with me to find the bed on the floor and things back to normal. This happened three times until the housefather would not come up to help me anymore. I only found out recently who had pulled this stunt.

Another way to relieve boredom was to join the wrestling team. Not only did this give one something to do in the afternoon, the girls loved the athletes, or so we thought. One of the downsides to being on the team was state weigh in, which occurred each December. In order to wrestle a certain weight class, it was necessary to be at that weight for weigh in. Of course, I was overweight and had to cut several pounds in just a three day period. This meant I ate nothing, drank little, and exercised a lot. I slept and attended classes in sweats and worked out every spare moment. The final day of state weigh in coincided with of our annual Christmas dinner and dance. I made weight one hour before the dinner. I had asked a girl to go, so I hurried back to the dorm, took a good shower, dressed in my best and only suit, and took her to dinner. This was a formal dinner, but I did not care! I was starved! I think I ate four plates of food that evening. I did not know it at the time, but I was allergic to turkey, which had been served. It makes me very sleepy, among other things. We left dinner and went to the dance. Since I had not slept much for three days, I was exhausted. The next thing I remember is my date shaking my arm and telling me it was time to leave. I don't think she had a good time.

ADVERTISING GENIUS

The school had a small canteen (snack bar), which was open a couple of evenings during the week. When I was in the eleventh grade, I, and a few of my friends, were selected to take the class that would qualify us to work there. Shortly after we all qualified, the RC Cola distributor dropped off several more cases of pop than the teacher/supervisor ordered. He made the fatal mistake of deciding to not have the extras picked up. Instead, he elected to give us a lesson in marketing strategy. We were given one simple task: find a way to move the extra product. "This is a great way for you to learn advertising strategy," he told us. We put our heads together and came up with a plan.

Our school athletic team name was the Rockets. It did not take us long to decide exactly what to do. It was simple! RC, ROCKET COLA! On the evening canteen was open, we had the announcement made at dinner that we had just received a shipment of a brand new product. You guessed it--ROCKET COLA. We knew that not many students drank RC Cola and would not recognize the shape of the bottle. Not only did we sell the overstock, we sold every bottle of RC in the place. The teacher arrived the next morning very pleased, until he learned just how we moved the product. After that, we received much instruction concerning ethics in advertising.

FAR-OUT FRIENDSHIPS

In spite of myself, I did develop some good friendships that lasted through high school, miraculously. One of those friends was Rob. His parents lived in Indianapolis. Since I did not get home very often, Rob's parents kind of adopted me. Every couple of months I spent the weekend with them. I got to know his mom, dad, and three sisters quite well. Rob's dad made a secret barbecue sauce that I can still taste! He worked for a major brand name food cannery as a product inspector, which gave him access to some of their special sauces. One particular summer day, he brought home a baby food sized jar of hot sauce. This was the exact measurement used for 100 gallons of chili beans. I could not wait to try it, loving spicy food.

"Dip the tip of a knife into it, wipe it off, and then briefly dip it into your soup," he told me.

I was tough! I plunged the knife into the jar and buried it in my bowl, showing off for Rob's oldest sister, who was fourteen, just like I. With a flourish, I scooped up a huge bite and shoved it into my mouth with gusto! Instantly, I could not breathe! My eyes didn't just water. I appeared to be weeping uncontrollably! Tears rushed from my eyes in a rage. My nose gushed mucus I had not yet formed, my throat closed up, and I could not say a word. I grabbed for my water glass, which Rob's dad grabbed away from me. Instead, he handed me a loaf of bread. "You will need this," he said, laughing.

I think I ate half of that loaf before I could talk again. Rob's dad laughingly told me how to treat the blisters I already had in my mouth and throat. I don't even want to write about the next day! By the way, Rob's sister thought I was an idiot. I really impressed her.

Another friend with whom I would hang out was Phil. We had been friends through our entire school experience. Since we were usually in the same dorm, there were often sibling rivalries that never lasted. There were times when, like brothers, we would fight over stupid things. Most of the time, we were involved in the same mischief, reading the same books, and, at times, interested in the same girl. This last interest would cause a friendly competition. The loser would congratulate the winner of the competition, and life went on. It is important to note that there were not that many eligible girls to pick from, so competition was high. Since there were not so many, it was important to walk a straight line. They all knew each other, and, if we were jerks, they all knew it and we didn't get a date for quite some time.

In spite of these rivalries, Phil and I spent quite a bit of time together during the summer following our tenth grade year. Since we did not live far apart in southern Indiana, and, since our folks were often glad to share us with the other set, we would spend a couple of weeks apart, and then our folks would arrange an opportunity for us to spend more time together. Wherever we were, we managed to have a great time.

We had moved to a small town, Adams, a "town" in name only. It was really a small group of homes with a combination post office and bar, a print shop, and an empty building that used to be a general store. Mom and Dad rented this building and converted the back third of it into living quarters for us. Since there was no plumbing inside, and since we did not have an outhouse, it was necessary to walk across the street to use the one behind the print shop. We became fast friends with the owners of that business! Dad eventually built an outhouse and placed it behind our building. I helped him dig the pit for it. It was a beautiful two-seater with a stand-up facility for the guys.

Mom had started an upholstery business, and decided to use the front of the building for that growing project. Before long, the local teenagers began hanging out in the shop because they had no place else to gather. Since Mom had teens of her own, and since she had a real love for teenagers, she converted half of the shop to a "recreation center". She put in a counter and sold snacks, soft drinks, and some basic grocery items. She contracted with a vendor and placed coin-operated games such as pinball, pool, and bowling, for the kid's entertainment. The teens would enter before school in the morning while awaiting the bus, purchase a pie or cake and a drink, and load up the jukebox and talk. It would get so loud at times that the bus driver would have to blow the horn several times before one of the teens would hear. They would rush out, leaving the music blaring, sometimes for an hour.

Phil and I had great times when he visited. We would purchase cigars and sit on the front porch like a couple of old men, waiting for some of the teenage guys to show up to smoke and talk with us. We would wait on the counter while Mom worked in the shop, or con some guy into taking us some place where we could get into some kind of mischief.

After a few days of that "fun", we were ready to move on to Phil's grandparents' home in North Vernon. Phil's grandfather had purchased a cabin near the Muscatatuck River. While nothing fancy, this place was wonderful! We could swim in the river or just loaf around under the shade trees in the yard.

This particular summer, Phil's mom and stepdad were living in the cabin. When I visited, his stepdad spent hours at the river with us. They also secured a couple of puppies for Phil, with which we bonded.

One particularly hot July night, we talked Phil's stepdad into letting us "camp out" in the back of his station wagon. We took our sleeping bags and a supply of food for munching out to the car, opened all of the windows and the back tailgate, and had a blast late into the night. When we finally drifted off to sleep, I was lying with my face to the driver's side of the car, with just barely enough room between me and the side to breathe. Phil lay on the other side with his back to the side of the car, facing the center. Sometime during the night, one of the puppies climbed into the car and lay down next to Phil, his nose nearly touching Phil's. I awoke to strange, loud utterances from Phil, which I have cleaned up since this is a family book. "Man, Sam! Your breath is awful! I would appreciate it if you would go back to your side of the car." I awoke out of my sleep, checked my surroundings, and began to laugh. Phil was not amused until he shook himself awake, checked his surroundings, and felt the location of the little dog. We both laughed so loud that his parents came out to see what was wrong. They got into the act, and we all stayed up for a while drinking lemonade and eating homemade cookies.

EVERY KID WANTS TO BE IN A BAND!

Later, a few of us at the school for the blind were introduced to some novelty instruments. In time, the "band" whittled down to four regulars. Rob played the saxophone, Mike played the guitar, Phil played the washtub bass, and I played the pogo cello, which was a metal oil can mounted on a flat stick. A spring was mounted on the bottom of the stick, which was bounced on a concrete stepping-stone. Snare drum wires were stretched across the front of the can and tightened until they vibrated when struck, producing a snare sound when struck with a wire brush. We practiced for hours! When we got what we considered to be pretty good, we chose a name and hit the road.

While Mom and Dad arranged the engagements and drove us, War on Poverty gathered a following as we toured southern Indiana and western Ohio, making our unusual music. We played auctions, festivals, family reunions, any place we could. We actually made money at it!

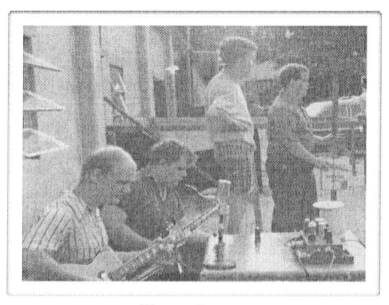

War on Poverty

There are many other things I could tell you, but I am not sure the statute of limitations has run out on some of those crimes. For instance, I know who removed the bolts from Rob's bed so that it fell down after he ran and jumped into it after sneaking off to the bathroom for a smoke in the middle of the night. I know who switched the salt and sugar in the Home Economics classroom. I know who kept stealing the skeleton out of the science room and putting it in strange places. But, I'm not telling. Well, maybe in a later book.

During all of this time keeping myself busy, I always felt that something was missing. While externally I appeared to have things together, internally I was falling apart. My life had no real meaning. I was not happy. There was no peace in my life. I was confused, angry, and frustrated with God because I thought He had deserted me.

CHAPTER 11

NOTHING TO LAUGH ABOUT

It was while I was in the sixth grade that I got the answer to my question, "Does Jesus love me?" Religious education at the school was limited to some brief instruction once a week during fourth and fifth grade, and brief services on Sunday for those who stayed over the weekend. God was taught in the abstract. He was never shown to be personally interested in any one individual. This only increased my confusion about His love and my blindness. I began to think that I was God's big joke, that I was only a good laugh for Him.

As Christmas vacation approached during my sixth grade year, I awaited the expected bus ticket for my transportation home. When it did not arrive, I became very concerned. The school would close down, and I needed some place to go. My parents did not have a phone, and there was no way to get in touch with them.

The Christmas program was over. School was officially out for the holiday season. I walked back to the dorm with the rest of the boys. Their chatter of excitement only brought me more grief. What was I going to do? The housemother had let me know in no uncertain terms that she was not going to be happy with me if she had to change her holiday plans to accommodate me. The last thing I wanted to do was make her unhappy.

As I walked into the dorm, Dad spoke to me and then gave me a big hug. Dad never hugged me unless someone was sick or had died, so I asked him, "Who is sick?"

"Nobody is sick."

"Who died?"

"Nobody. Come with me."

I was very happy that my housemother was happy, but I did not understand Dad at all! As we drove off the campus Dad began to sing. He was not singing the songs I expected. He was singing hymns! That was the last thing I wanted to hear! I rolled down the car window and plunged my head out into the freezing wind as it rushed by the speeding car. After a few seconds, I pulled my head inside and asked Dad what was going on. He told me that he had accepted Christ that past Sunday at a new church the family was attending.

I figured I could put up with Dad as long as no one else had gotten religion. When I walked into the house, I immediately noticed a different atmosphere. It seemed that every person in that house had lost his or her mind!

I went to church out of obligation the following Sunday. I cannot tell you what the pastor said during his sermon. All I can tell you is that when he gave the invitation, I was the first out of my seat and at the altar. All at once I began to understand. For the first time in my life, I began to feel that Jesus really loved me. I felt things would be different. I was about to face some shocking reality.

As I knelt at that altar and received Christ into my life, I was filled with happiness and other emotions that I could never describe. It was so exciting to realize that Jesus really loved me! But what about the second question I had asked my mother years before: "Why did God make me blind?" While I was excited about the realization that God loved me, I was puzzled about the fact that I was still blind. Then the pastor said something that got me even more excited. "Now that Sammy has accepted Christ, he is going to get his sight."

It was all going to happen for me! Now that Christ loved me, I was going to be able to see! No more would

I be God's big joke! I could not wait! I would have done anything that pastor asked me to do at that moment.

However, I did not expect what happened next. It seemed that the entire congregation rushed to the front of that little church. They crowded around me, placing their hands on my body. I was terrified. They all began praying loudly, at once. They slapped me, shook me, and commanded the demon of blindness to come out of me. The pastor had his hands over my eyes and continually shook my head violently. This went on for about ten minutes.

Finally, everything was silent. Everyone went back to their seats, and I was alone in the front of the church with the pastor, his hands over my eyes. He removed his hands and I was still blind. I cannot relate how disappointed I was! I knelt there crying, broken and frustrated. "You just didn't have enough faith," the pastor told me. I did not even know about faith. How was I supposed to have it?

In the course of the next year, I was prayed for countless times. Each time I was not healed, I was ridiculed and shamed for not having enough faith. I did everything I was told to increase my faith: I stayed up all night several nights praying for faith; I fasted and prayed; I shared my newfound faith in Christ at school and was beaten by my roommates for it. Yet I still "did not have enough faith."

After a year, some of the church leaders came to our home and asked my parents that we not attend that church anymore. The excuse was given that our clothes were not good enough, but I have always felt that it was because of my "lack of faith". We were not the worst dressed family in the church. I became bitter towards God. If these were Christians, if they represented the loving God they kept telling me about, I wanted nothing to do with them, or God.

At the age of twelve, I began to listen to my teachers at school who told me that God, if there was a God, was inside a person. All one needed to do was look inside and find him. I began to look inside and found only loneliness and emptiness. The deeper I looked, the worse I felt. I turned to organizations to find relief, organizations like the Boy Scouts and DeMolay. They offered me nothing of substance. I would feel good for a while, and then I would feel worse.

At times, I would give God a cursory glance. One of these times was when I was about seventeen. I asked the campus pastor about salvation after one of his Sunday morning services. He assured me that someone would talk to me about that subject. The next day, I was summoned to the school psychologist's office and ridiculed for my delusions. I was eventually put into psychiatric counseling for my religious delusions.

When my parents moved the family to Florida in 1972, I willingly went with them even though I had only one more semester of my senior year at the Indiana School for the Blind. I thought that maybe a new location would mean a new start. I ditched all that I knew, and my friends, and set off on a new adventure. Within two weeks of moving, I knew that things were just the same. I had brought all that I was with me. Even though my location had changed, I had not. Now I was not only sick of my life, I was even sicker of my circumstances. I had moved from a school where I was somebody to a public school where I was, at best, a novelty. I moved from a class of fourteen, where I was senior class president, to a senior class where I was not even part of the crowd.

Before long I found a crowd to be a part of, but it was the wrong crowd. A member of the senior class discovered that I played the bass guitar and approached me, asking if I would like to jam with him some time. Of course, I agreed. That very evening, after I had gone to bed, he showed up at my house. I got dressed and went with him. He played a mean guitar, if you like acid rock, which I did! We played almost all night, quitting in time to get ourselves together for school. Within a week, I was the bass player for his band. I quickly got absorbed into that culture and the activities that went along with it. My search for artificial means of peace only brought me more unhappiness. I became depressed and paranoid, and I started having suicidal thoughts. I was bottoming out! Little did I know that, although it would take almost three years for me to see it, God was throwing me a lifeline.

Rev. Walter Rollins (his real name) was right there to help my parents unload the truck when they pulled in with our few possessions from Indiana. He was the pastor of the Hilliard Alliance Church (now, First Alliance Church of Hilliard). This small Christian and Missionary Alliance church would play a great part in my life. It was through this church, particularly this man, that God would begin to extend that lifeline to me.

"Brother Rollins" was an ex-marine. Although he stood six feet five inches, I discovered that he was the gentlest man I would ever know. As I stood beside the truck that day, wondering where to begin, he climbed into it and grabbed the kitchen stove, the oven of which Mom had loaded with homemade canned goods, and carried it off by himself. As he passed me he asked, without pausing for an answer, "Will I see you in church on Sunday?"

I said yes for two reasons. I was not about to say no to someone who could single-handedly carry a kitchen stove that Mom had packed off the truck, and I wanted to impress my three female cousins who attended the church. Little did I know that at that very moment God was putting things in place that would impact my life for eternity.

I would party on Saturday night, and go to church on Sunday morning. As soon as church was over, I would rush home, get out of my dress clothes and party until bedtime. On Monday I was off to school, and the cycle would start over.

Brother Rollins started showing up where I was. Not once did he condemn my lifestyle. He kept loving me, and, when I let him, sharing Scriptural principles with me. I tried everything in my power for two years to get rid of him, to no avail. Then one day I hit on à plan that I was sure would work.

The Rollins family had moved 11 miles south to the town of Callahan to start a church there. The new church needed some tables and chairs. Since I had started a used furniture store, I contributed all they needed, thinking that this good deed would get the preacher to leave me alone! It didn't work. Instead, he invited me to attend and see what had been done with my gift of kindness. The service I attended "turned out" to be an evangelistic service. I left that service angry and frustrated.

I decided that the only way I was going to get rid of this pest was to "get saved." Since I had been in the drama club at school and was a pretty good actor, and, since I had a working knowledge of the Bible, thanks to Brother Rollins, I decided that I would just have to "get saved!"

I practiced until I got it right and showed up at church. At the end of the service I was right up front at the prayer rail. I said all of the right things. I even cried. Convinced that my commitment was genuine, Brother Rollins and the small congregation, which included my Mom and Dad, rejoiced. I went home rejoicing that day as well, but for another reason. I thought I had finally hit on the solution to get the preacher off my back so that I could live my life without embarrassment or conviction.

My problem got even larger. Brother Rollins decided that I needed to be discipled. Not only was he showing up even more, he was admonishing me, correcting me, and using the Bible to point me in the direction I had said I wanted to go. Unable to tell him no, I found myself not showing up for band practices and parties in order to attend some church meeting. My friends began to call me a fanatic and drifted away.

In 1974 I agreed to attend a men's retreat with Brother Rollins. I am still not sure how this came about. On the weekend of the retreat our band was to audition for a club job. Instead of attending the audition, I went to the retreat. During a missionary slide presentation, I truly surrendered my life to Christ and rededicated myself to Him. At that very moment I knew I was called into ministry. I turned and whispered this fact to my pastor. "Great," he said. "You are preaching on Sunday evening."

My first sermon was so boring, I yawned! I destroyed John 3:16! As I walked off of the platform, Brother Rollins approached me. "That was terrible! You are preaching again next Sunday." And preach I did. After several attempts, I was at least able to keep people awake.

When we arrived back at our cabin at the retreat, I picked up the single volume of the Braille Bible I had brought with me for show. I had not even checked to see which volume it was. Since I knew that Christians were supposed to read their Bibles, I opened it and randomly placed my finger on a Braille line. "And the peace of God which passeth all understanding shall keep your hearts and minds through Christ Jesus." (Philippians 4:7, King James Version). That was what I had been looking for all of my life! There it was right under my fingers!

"God, please give me that peace," I prayed. "You promised."

I went to sleep that night expecting to wake the next morning with an endless feeling of euphoria. I awoke feeling no different than I had when I fell asleep. Were God's promises a lie, or had I just imagined that I had read a promise that I could receive what I wanted, what I now knew I needed?

For nearly three years after this, I struggled with self-doubt, questioning if God really loved me. He had not given me my vision, He had not given me peace, I still struggled with old lifestyle issues, and an incredible sense of loneliness and insecurity. Then, in a moment, during the most tragic event in my life, God opened my eyes to the truth through a robin's song.

I was a student at Toccoa Falls College in northeast Georgia on the morning of November 6, 1977. When the earthen dam holding back a large lake above the Falls gave way early that morning, all of our lives were changed forever. When all was over, 39 people were dead. Parts of the campus were destroyed or rendered unusable by the millions of gallons of water. Early that morning I had walked Muffin and headed back up the stairs to enter the girl's dorm to which we had all been evacuated. Before entering, I stopped at the top of the stairs on the porch and leaned against a large pillar. My heart cried out to God as I prayed the same prayer I had uttered at least a hundred times that morning. "God, why?"

As I stood there praying this simple prayer, a robin flew to the roof over my head and began to sing as the sun came up. The cool morning breeze blew the stench of death, raw sewage, and destruction into my face, God spoke to my heart. It was as though God said to me, "This robin may have been on that hillside when the dam broke. Maybe she lost her tree home, her mate, her young ones. Yet, in spite of this, she flies to a pinnacle overlooking the destruction and performs the task I created her to do. She sees past the destruction. She sees the beauty of the world I created, and sings to greet the new day."

It was then that I began to understand the "peace of God". It is not a giddy happiness or contrived joy. Rather, it is a confidence that God is in control of every life situation and that He has my best interest in mind. "God," I said, "I want that peace." And He gave me that peace! Finally, I began to understand the extent of God's love for me and that He couldn't care less that I was blind. God had made me blind for a purpose. He wanted to use me, not in spite of my disability, but because of it. I realized that God was not laughing at me. He never had been. I was filled with such joy! At that moment, my whole perspective on life changed. Finally, I really knew there was something to laugh about.

CHAPTER 12

LOVE IS BLIND AND KIND OF STUPID

Since I attended a school for the blind all but one semester of my formative education, I had plenty of experience dating blind and partially-sighted girls. The school was small, so we all knew each other too well. This both simplified and complicated dating. You broke up with a girl and every other girl on the campus knew it within minutes (and this *before* social media!). You couldn't get another date until some other guy became a worse cad than you and your antics were forgotten. I learned to live with these social arrangements and got along quite well.

That all changed when my family moved from Indiana to Florida my last semester of high school. I was plunked down in a public school where everyone was sighted. There were no more blind girls to date. The "sighted world" was quite different. I resolved, however, that I was not going to go dateless, especially during my senior year of high school.

One girl caught my eye. We will call her Megan. Megan was pretty, witty, and, I thought, interested in me. There were lots of other guys who also found her to be pretty, witty, and interested in them. The problem was that I lacked confidence to ask her out on a date. I knew that if I stood any chance in the world, I would have to screw up my courage and ask her out. I stayed in my room one entire weekend practicing just what I would say to her. I prepared a most eloquent speech, one that I was sure would sweep her off her feet and make her pledge to be mine forever!

I met her in front of her locker in the hall of the school on Monday morning, informed her that I had something important to ask her, and made my speech. For thirty seconds or so after I finished, she just stood there looking at me. I did not know what to think. I could not see her facial expression. Was she moved? Was she afraid? Was she going to throw up? Then she started laughing. That was not the result I had hoped for! "You know," she said, "it would be a lot easier to take you seriously if you did not have that booger hanging out of your nose."

Somehow I was never able to overcome that image. I went dateless my senior year. In fact, I went pretty much dateless for several years after that. My confidence was shaken. I could not be around a member of the opposite sex without checking my nose. My next serious date was three years after I got out of high school.

I met Doreen at the church in Orlando where I was serving as a pastoral intern in 1975. She had stopped by to see the pastor about some matter and he introduced us. He was hoping she could convince me to attend Toccoa Falls College where she would begin attending in the fall of the next year. I was not convinced right away, but the girl intrigued me. All of my inhibitions left me. I asked her out, and she agreed to go.

Immediately after she agreed to go out with me, my self-confidence waned. I confided to my friend Jack, the associate pastor, my concerns. "What you need to do," he said, "is to take her some place nice, some place where you can talk. It needs to be some place elegant, but not expensive. The place you need to take her is Ireland's downtown."

I trusted him implicitly! The next Saturday night, Doreen picked me up in her Gremlin (yes, a Gremlin!). We bought a dollar's worth of gasoline, which gave us a couple of gallons, and we were off to our romantic evening.

Ireland's was anything but romantic! We walked into a smoke-filled room. The noise level was deafening! There was a musician, if you could call him that, belting out his performance through a distorted sound system. People were shouting to each other over his "performance." "Do you want to leave?" I asked. "No," she said. "Let's eat. I'm starved!"

We received the menu and she shouted the offerings to me along with their prices. I guess Jack and I had a different idea of the word "expensive." I checked my wallet, figured out what I could do, and explained to Doreen the benefits of chopped beef steak. At that, I knew that I was going to have to stiff the waiter, which got easier to do as the night wore on.

Doreen and I walked out into the night air, breathed it in gratefully and decided to call it an early evening. I had just enough money left to get us across the toll road and back to the church. I was supposed to meet the pastor at midnight to deliver the sermon I was to preach the next morning. He had the interns practice on him the first time we preached. He would offer his critique and we had the rest of the night to correct our mistakes before our morning delivery. It was about eleven when we left the restaurant. I figured that it would take about thirty minutes to get across Orlando. That would give me fifteen minutes to repair the effects of this lousy evening and maybe get a second date with Doreen.

So much for my calculations. I discovered that a dollar's worth of gasoline does not take a Gremlin as far as I expected. We ran out of gas on the toll road between Ireland's and the church, which was on the east side of Orlando. If this happened today, we would not have a problem. However, it was quite different in Orlando in

1975. There was absolutely no one on the road that late, even on a Saturday night! Most red-blooded American guys would have loved this situation. Most would fake a situation like this, but I knew two things: first of all, if I had anything like "this" in mind, Doreen would surely not be interested, especially after the evening I had just given her; secondly, I knew that the pastor would be waiting for me, and that he would not buy the "We ran out of gas" story. At twelve-thirty, a policeman showed up with a gas can, and we were on our way. The pastor did not buy my story!

Doreen and I dated off and on for three years after that eventful evening. Our relationship terminated finally when I met Ann.

LEARNING TO LOVE

My relationship with Doreen was quite rocky. I never seemed to get this relationship thing quite right. I never really felt accepted. My self-confidence waxed and waned. I was lonely and convinced that I was destined to be that way for the rest of my life.

In October of 1975, I moved back home to north Florida and began to sort out what I was going to do about my ministerial training. In January of 1976, I began to take classes at Luther Rice Seminary in Jacksonville. It did not take long for me to realize that I would need some good readers.

The youth pastor at the Baptist church down the road from us placed an advertisement in their newsletter notifying the teenagers that a blind college student needed a few good readers. Kathryn was one of the teens that responded. When I called her to set up an appointment to talk about the possibility of her reading for me, I noticed that she got more and more quiet as we conversed on the phone. We set the date and time, and she arrived at my parents' home right on time. I was impressed!

Our home was small. There was barely enough room for all of us, not to mention my new need for a study. I had designated a part of my bedroom for this purpose. In my mind, that was what that part of the room was used for. The fact that there was a bed in the room had slipped my mind. I was going to use that room for study, and study only, while readers were present. Without giving it a second thought, I ushered Kathryn into the room and closed the door to keep my younger brothers out. I pointed to the desk chair, and, without giving it a second thought, sat down on the bed and leaned back luxuriously to interview this possible reader.

"Can we open the door?" she asked. And then it hit me. I had, without any forethought, asked this young, pretty girl into my room! I spent the next several minutes apologizing, making the matter worse.

This situation was worsened by Kathryn's first impression of me. You see, she had seen me before! As stated previously, I had joined an acid rock band as their bass player. We were not especially good, but we were loud and rebellious. When we "performed" at a talent show put on by the county school system, my friends and I terrified a middle school aged Kathryn. The fact that we were thrown off the stage by the teachers in charge did not help to pacify her fears. When I called her to set up the appointment and identified who I was, she recognized me and was terrified! I had failed to tell her of my rededication to Christ, and the advertisement in the newsletter did not state that I was pursuing a Bible college education.

As Kathryn got over her fear of me, our friendship began to grow and flourish. I discovered a person who was warm, charming, and accepting. She was the type of girl I always hoped I would meet! The frustrating thing for me was that neither of us had any interest in developing a dating relationship. Instead, we became the best of friends. When Ann and I began to date, Kathryn became Ann's friend also. In fact, she was very instrumental in getting us together. Kathryn was the first person who truly accepted me as I was. She showed me what it meant to care for someone unconditionally, to love selflessly. She prepared me to meet the love of my life.

THE ROAD TO ANN

In the summer of 1977, I proposed to Doreen, and she said she would marry me. I moved to Toccoa Falls College, partially to be near her, but also because God was leading me there. Shortly after I arrived on campus, Doreen left. She dropped out of college and returned home to Orlando. By October, our letters got fewer and fewer, yet it seemed that neither of us wanted to face the inevitable.

In the summer of 1978, while bicycle riding with brothers Dale and Tim, I had an accident (I didn't learn my lesson years before), fracturing my elbow, necessitating the removal of my right radial head. The surgery resulted in some nerve damage, which made my right hand virtually unusable for several months. Since it was necessary for me to use that hand for taking Braille notes, I dropped out of college for a semester to allow my arm to heal.

I could not stay away from the school, however. I loved and missed the students I had met. I loved and missed the area. It was shortly after Thanksgiving that a friend and I made a trip to Toccoa. She went to check out the college, and I to see my friends. While visiting with one of my friends in the center of campus, a shy, pretty girl came out of the dorm in front of us and headed over to the snack bar for her afternoon shift. My friend whistled and spoke to her. He introduced us, and I said, "I would have whistled also, but I did not want to leave a bad first impression." I found out some time later that Ann was quite impressed with that statement. She even told her parents about our meeting.

I returned to school the next semester. Ann was in a couple of my classes. As we got acquainted, we did not care much for each other. Ann thought I was obnoxious, and I thought she was a snob. As it turns out, Ann was just shy.

The professor who taught one of the classes we both attended had a custom of asking students to share any concerns they had before beginning his class. We would then pray about those concerns. One particular morning, I shared my burden to minister to people with disabilities. Ann was intrigued by what I had shared, but she said nothing to me, at least not immediately. We did not talk to each other unless it was necessary. This all changed a few days later.

My relationship with God was really growing during this time. One thing he had shown me was that I needed to end my relationship with Doreen. I wrote a letter to her stating that the relationship was not good for either of us and that I wanted out. On a cold February afternoon, I put on my jacket, slipped the letter into my pocket and left my dorm room headed for the post office. As I walked up the hill toward the center of the campus, I was praying about direction for my life without Doreen in it. After I dropped the letter into the mail slot, I headed towards the Eagles' Nest (the campus snack bar) for a cup of hot chocolate. As I approached the door, God impressed on my heart that I was to minister to the first person that spoke to me after I entered. "All right Lord," I said, "whatever you want."

"Hi, Sam," Ann said from behind the counter. I literally stepped back a step or two. I ordered my hot chocolate, intending to sit at a table as far away from Ann as possible. I was not willing to "minister" to this one! As I paid for my beverage, a mutual friend came in to ask Ann if she would work part of his shift that evening so that he could play intramural basketball. I made a mental note to avoid the Eagles' Nest that evening. I got out of there after some casual conversation, feeling quite smug that I had not committed any mistakes that would necessitate getting involved in this girl's life past this level.

That evening I had my dinner in the cafeteria and headed back to my room for some serious study time. About two hours later, I felt an urgent need to go to the post office and mail that letter I had written to Doreen. I slipped on my jacket and headed for the center of campus. When I got to the post office, I put my hand in my pocket, and remembered that I had already mailed the letter that afternoon. It was bitterly cold that evening, so I thought that I would go get a cup of hot chocolate. I reasoned that the Eagle's Nest would be crowded, and that, if Ann was still working, she would be much too busy for any conversation. I was right! The place was crowded. I got my beverage and proceeded to the table farthest away from the counter. I hurriedly finished my chocolate and proceeded to leave. Friend after friend detained me. Finally, I heard Ann's replacement arrive, and I made a beeline for the door. "Are you going to leave without saying goodbye?" It was Ann's voice. "Goodbye," I said, and put my hand on the door. "Wait, I need to talk to you," she said.

I was hooked. There was no way out without being rude. We walked over to a table and sat down. We made small talk for a while, and then she asked if we could go somewhere quiet so that we could talk. That was the last thing I wanted to do, but I was already in this far. We found a quiet place, and she told me that she was interested in the burden for ministry I had shared in class. I shared more with her about the ministry God had placed on my heart, feeling that this could not hurt. After all, it would be good to have someone praying for me. When she told me that she wanted to help me get a ministry started, I was taken aback!

"You know," I said, "if we are going to start a ministry together, we have to at least like each other. I think we should pray about our friendship." She agreed. We prayed right then and there, and God began healing the ill feelings. As we prayed over the next couple of months, God did more than heal our friendship. He began to give us deeper feelings than friendship for each other. Two months later, we were an item and the ministry was established.

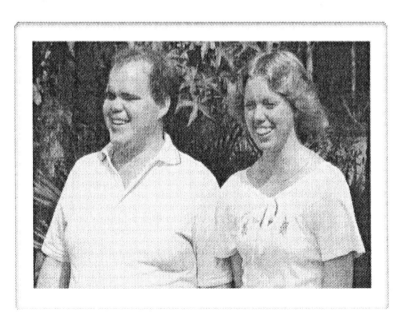

OUR FIRST OFFICIAL DATE

The Dillard House is one of those places where you pay one price and make a pig of yourself! I had been there a couple of times and knew the food was good. I asked Ann and one of our friends to go there with me. I asked the friend to go along since it was some distance from the college and she had a car. Ann had not brought her car with her that semester. We ate our fill and the check was presented to me. When Ann read the total, I almost passed out. The price had gone up considerably since I had last been there. No matter how I stretched the dollars in my pocket, I was short! I borrowed from both Ann and our friend to get out of the restaurant. I was certain that would be our last date, but it wasn't.

Our dates were usually simple. We would take a walk in a park or take a trip to Helen, Georgia, a Swiss Alpine-style village near Toccoa. Since I obviously did not have much money, it was necessary to get creative. It was on one of these simple dates that Ann informed me that God had shown her we were going to get married. I obviously believed her.

I had forgotten that I owed Ann money from our first date. She reminded me in quite an unusual way. It was the end of the semester, and Mom and Dad arrived to take me home for the summer. Since Ann had not spent much time with them, and I wanted them to get to know her a little better, I asked her to join us for a quick lunch before we left town. She agreed to go. We had a pleasant lunch, and I paid the bill. This time I had money. No sooner had the cashier given me my change than Ann snatched it out of my hand. "That's mine," she said. Dad asked me in a stage whisper, "What are you paying for?" Ann informed my parents how her new cheapskate boyfriend didn't even have enough money to get out of the restaurant on our first date. Mom informed her that it was not going to get much better. I had always been, and would always be, a cheapskate. I am sure glad Ann knew she was kidding!

MEETING ANN'S FAMILY

As our relationship grew Ann told me more about her family. She had only one sister, who was a year younger. I actually got a chance to meet Leah one weekend. She and Ann, along with a cousin and another friend attended a Christian night at an amusement park in Atlanta. The girls accompanied Ann back to the dorm for the night. The next day was Easter, so we all attended the sunrise service together. Leah did not say much to me, so I was unable to form any impression.

Along with summer break came an invitation from Ann to spend a week with her at her parents' farm. I accepted the invitation with some reservation. I arrived scared to death! Ann says that it was the only time she saw me without much to say and without any appetite.

The one thing that Ann neglected to tell me about her sister was that she liked to hunt the doves that would congregate in the pasture. The first evening I was at her home, sitting quietly in the living room after dinner, I felt cold steel on my neck. Leah had placed the barrel of her shotgun on my shoulder. I was not sure what was happening. My heart was literally in my throat! They all had a good laugh at my expense.

"YOU HAVE TO ASK MY PARENTS"

Even though Ann had told me that we were going to get married, I felt that it was necessary to ask her. I did so and she said yes. "You have to ask my parents," she told me. I thought, "What could be so hard about that?"

I will never forget that hot summer afternoon. I sat in Ann's parents' living room. Ann sat beside me on the couch, and her mother was seated in a chair to our left. Her father was outside, working somewhere on the property. I took a breath and asked, "What would you think about Ann and me getting married?"

I should have said something like, "Ann and I would like to get married." Or I should have asked, "May I marry your daughter?" I chose to ask her what she thought. Her answer was not exactly what I wanted to hear. "You will have to ask Papa."

Shortly after my question and her answer, Ann's mother left the room. "That was not the way to ask," Ann said. I agreed. You would think I learned a lesson. Judge for yourself.

That entire evening, I was incredibly nervous. I was wondering when the time would come, when it would be right to "ask Papa". I went to bed that night with feelings of both regret and relief. I knew there would not be time to do the asking the next day. Ann was taking me for my first visit to Walt Disney World for my birthday. We would be too busy. Or so I thought.

The next morning we were eating a hasty breakfast before heading off for our two-hour ride to Disney. I was kind of relieved that Ann and I would have a pleasant day alone, time to recover from my botched conversation with her mother.

I was thinking how especially good my scrambled eggs were when Ann's mom said, "Why don't you ask Papa the question you asked me yesterday afternoon?" I had just taken a bite of eggs and just about swallowed my fork! Being raised to respect my elders and do exactly as I was told, I hurriedly swallowed the bite of eggs and blurted out, "What would you think about Ann and me getting married?"

I was nearly twenty-five years old. I knew that he was the father of a daughter. I knew that it did not take a rocket scientist to figure out what any father thought about his daughter getting married. I also knew by Ann's comment that that was not a good way to ask her parents if we could get married, but Ann's mom suggested that I ask "the question", so I asked!

He put down his fork and looked at me for what seemed like an eternity. I sat, sweating, thinking about the thousand or so other ways I could have asked that question. I wondered what Ann would say and do if he said no. I wondered what I would do. I wondered if we were going to Disney after all, or if I would be catching a train back to Jacksonville with a one-way ticket.

Finally his answer came, slowly, deliberately. "If you feel like it is the Lord's will, well…" He NEVER finished that sentence. Ann and I figured that since he did not say no, we could proceed with our plans, and proceed we did.

MAKING AN "ASS" OF MYSELF

We had a great day at Disney World. As we walked down Main Street, USA, I told Ann I wanted to find a little something for her mother. I think I was looking for a way to make up for the lousy question I asked her. We stepped into one of the shops, and there it was! Ann's mom really likes Eeyore from the Winnie the Pooh stories. The glass Eeyore seemed to jump out at me shouting, "Buy me. She will love me!" So I bought him.

Later that evening I presented the glass donkey to Ann's mother with this statement: "Here. I saw this and it made me think of you." She held the statue, looked at it and said, "What does that mean?" My face turned redder than I think it ever had. Twice in two days!!! Mom once told me that it was a miracle I could talk at all around that foot in my mouth. Ann's mom looked at me and laughed. "It's okay," she said. "I think, at least, I hope, I know what you mean." She still has that donkey.

SCORE ONE FOR THE TURKEY

At college, it seemed to be almost impossible to keep the secret about when a girl was going to get her engagement ring. Usually the girl's roommate would find out, she would tell her best friend, and... I decided that the date I was going to give Ann her ring was going to be my secret, well, mine and one other trusted friend's. Of course, I earned his trust by threatening his life.

In order to protect the sanctity of the moment, I told Ann's roommate a lie. I gave her the wrong date. She bought it, and, although she promised not to tell a single soul, told her best friend who told someone else and... The end result was that someone let it slip to Ann that she was going to get her engagement ring real soon. Ann was furious with me, as I knew she would be. She fumed and I smiled, which made her fume even more.

On the designated evening, I insisted that we take a walk so that we could work out our little problem. We walked up to the cemetery on campus and sat on an old bench. I reached into my pocket and produced the ring. By this time, I think she had heard of the false date for the big event. She was blown away! I waited patiently for her emotional response.

"You turkey!" she cried, smacking me on the arm. Apparently she got over the anger. She married me anyway. I think she likes turkey!

HERE COMES THE GROOM

We were married in Ann's home church on Father's Day, June 15, 1980. I am not sure Ann's father was pleased with her gift to him that particular year. Two weeks before we were married, I took the train from Jacksonville to Ann's hometown to help with the preparations, and to spend time with my future in-laws. Since the rehearsal dinner and reception were going to be in Ann's parents' home, there was quite a bit to do to get ready. In the midst of all the manual labor, I ended up being paired with my soon-to-be sister-in-law, Leah, for some projects. Ann's mother was working alongside us. Trying to break the ice, I asked, "You know the story of Jacob. He worked seven years for Rachel and ended up with Leah. Is this going to happen to me?" Leah looked at me and said, "Not a chance!" I guess I knew where I stood.

The wedding day finally arrived. Since the wedding was on a Sunday, we got up, went to church, came back to Ann's parents' home, had lunch, and went to get married. A typical Sunday afternoon.

I have never been so nervous in my entire life. This nervousness was due partially to the fact that Dale was my best man. I never knew what he was going to pull. And pull something he did. Upon hearing our musical cue to enter the sanctuary, the pastor opened the door, and we started out to the front of the church. As we were leaving the room, Dale asked one of the other groomsmen, "Are you going out there? If you are going, I'm not." "Well," the groomsman said, "if you are going I'm not." We left them arguing behind us. They both showed up with big smiles on their faces.

The wedding went off without a hitch. Well, almost. We had asked Brother Rollins to officiate the ceremony, with the assistance of Ann's pastor. It was a simple, God-honoring ceremony, with vows that fit us to a tee. Brother Rollins had everything written down in a little book, from which he read, with the exception of one of the prayers, which was not scripted. As was his custom, when it came time to pray, he closed his book and bowed his head, forgetting to keep his finger in the place where he left off. At the conclusion of his prayer, he opened the book, and began fumbling through the pages to find his place. The pause, and the silence, seemed eternal! Since he didn't know what to do, he looked at me and said, "Kiss your bride." Even though that wasn't the right place in the ceremony, and because I felt sorry for him, and to give him time to find his place, I obliged his instructions with a long, passionate kiss. Feeling like we were being watched (we were, not only by everyone in the church, which was full, but by Brother Rollins as well), we ended our kiss and once again waited for him to find his place in the book.

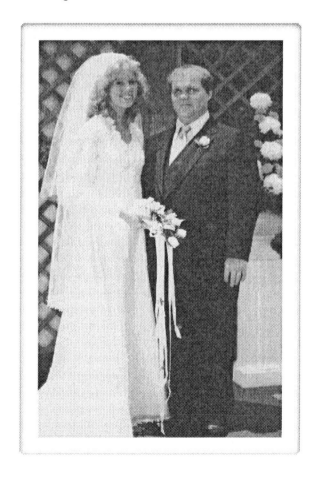

Maybe I am an incurable romantic, but I always wondered what would be the first thing my wife said to me after we took our vows and were headed up the aisle toward the back of the church. I will never forget the first words of my new wife. After Brother Rollins pronounced us husband and wife and introduced us to the congregation, we joined hands and headed toward the back of the church. My heart was racing with anticipation as I awaited the soft romantic voice of my new wife. What would she say first? Would it be, "Hi, Husband" or "I love you?" Would she whisper something I would blush to repeat to anyone else, but cherish for the rest of my life? I waited, and then the words came, words I will never forget: "I'm hungry!"

Ann had not eaten much the couple of weeks before we were married. It seemed that when the anxiety and busyness surrounding the wedding were behind her she was ready to make up for lost time. "Are you going to eat that?" became her favorite question during our honeymoon.

OPEN INVITATION

As I stated earlier, the reception was held at Ann's parents' home. On that day, their house was overflowing with well-wishers, so much so that the front door was seldom closed. This gave a feeling of welcome to all. One guest was neither invited nor expected, but he came anyway. We did not discover him until we were looking at the pictures several weeks later. The wedding cake was a beautiful multi-tiered one, decorated with purple violets, Ann's chosen flower for the wedding. A close look at the cake photograph reveals a fly confidently perched on the top tier. You can almost see a big smile on its little fly face.

THAT HONEYMOON FEELING

Usually, the bride and groom are the first to leave the reception. That was not the case for us. We were the last to leave. Ann's sister had agreed to take us to where the car was hidden. It was necessary to hide the car because Dale was there. We also left late because we wanted to be sure certain out-of-town guests, especially Dale, were well on their way home before we started on our way. We did not want to be followed.

It was about five in the evening when we finally got on our way. We were headed to Lakeland, about sixty miles away, where Ann had reserved a room for us. On the way, we decided to attend a church in a small town where Ann knew the pianist. Ann, being raised to be a good Baptist girl, was not about to miss church. We quietly slipped in and took our seats. The two elderly ladies behind us noticed us right away. "You aren't from here, are you?" one of the matrons asked Ann. "No," she said. "We just got married this afternoon and are on our way to our honeymoon." The lady looked at us with wonder. "Honey," she said to Ann incredulously, "if I had just gotten married, I sure wouldn't be in church!"

We left the church and stopped for an evening meal before heading to the hotel. After finally arriving late that evening, we enjoyed a wonderful first night as husband and wife, rising the next morning and heading off to our honeymoon destination. Being poor college students, we were strapped financially, so I arranged with some friends to use their guest cottage. The "cottage" was a renovated metal barn. It had been fixed up quite nicely. The cottage was located in the middle of nowhere. It was not air conditioned, and it was June in Florida. But we did not mind too much.

The week flew, and before we knew it, it was time to head back home to Toccoa, Georgia to settle into our new apartment together. On the way back home, we stopped at my parents' to spend a couple of days. My sister Jane was there with her four kids, the youngest being two years old, and one of my sister Susan's daughters. They had all come down for the wedding and had spent the week with my parents. As we were leaving to head back to Georgia, I made a mistake for which I am not sure I have ever been forgiven. Jane was also getting ready to leave. In saying goodbye to Mom and Dad, she commented that she was dreading the long trip back to Indiana. I picked the wrong time to be polite. "Why don't you stop by our place for a couple of days? You could break up the trip, and Ann could get to know you and the kids."

She took me up on my offer. It was a long, quiet trip to Toccoa with Jane and her station wagon full of kids following closely behind us. When we arrived home to our small one bedroom apartment, the one with the bathroom you got to by going through our bedroom, I explained to all of our guests that I was going to carry my new wife over the threshold. I had picked her up gingerly to carry her into the home, when we heard a tiny voice behind us exclaim, "Mommy, I gotta' pee!" Needless to say, our first couple of days in our new home were unusual.

After Jane and the crowd left, we began to settle into our home. We had no idea how God was going to use that place, and us, during that next year to provide a place of comfort. The year we were married, one of the missionaries-in-residence at the college died from cancer. His widow and children remained on campus at the college. The fourteen-year-old girl bonded with Ann and me almost immediately after we invited her to stop by after school. She became like one of the family. Her mother would call us to inquire if her daughter was with us, and she usually was. It was then that we discovered that our life would always have young people in it.

The first day Grace (her real name) came by to visit us after school, she got involved with our wedding album. As she looked through the pictures, she looked up at me and asked innocently, "So, what did you do on your honeymoon?" I thought nothing of the question, but she sure did. She blushed as only a fourteen-year-old girl can. Several years later after she married, I asked her innocently, "So, what did you do on your honeymoon?" She blushed again.

CHAPTER 13

THE EYES HAVE IT

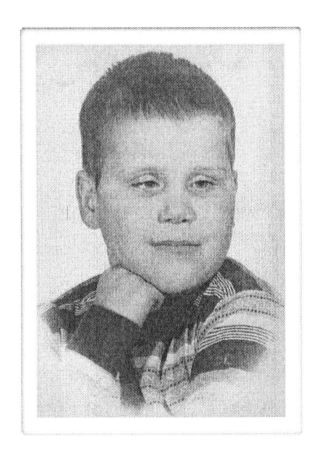

I think Ann fell in love with my eyes before she fell in love with the rest of me. When we started dating she would often comment about my beautiful blue eyes. All I knew about my eyes was that they hurt most of the time. I had been to a number of doctors who had diagnosed the problem as one thing or another, but had never provided a solution for the pain.

In 1984, four years after we were married, I began experiencing severe pain in my right eye, so severe that I could not stand it. We found an ophthalmologist who diagnosed the problem, but did nothing for it. He seemed to feel that I was exaggerating the pain level. Two days after visiting him, my right eye began to swell and throb. Ann called for a follow-up visit and was informed that the doctor was playing golf and had no intention of being disturbed. She asked for a referral from the receptionist and got one. We visited that doctor's office that afternoon. Fourteen hours later, I was on the operating table having my right eye removed.

I was psychologically unprepared for this surgery. I did not realize how much I took the light perception I had in that eye for granted. When it was removed, I really missed the ability to see whether a light was on or off, or whether it was a sunny or cloudy day. I soon adjusted, however, and the fun began.

I will never forget the day I was fitted with my first prosthetic eye. Since my health insurance company was paying for it, they elected to have me fitted with a stock eye, not one that was made for my socket. It was interesting to sit in a room with a man who had a cabinet filled with literally hundreds of eyes of various sizes, colors, and shapes. We tried out eyes for about twenty minutes until we found one that fit reasonably well, and reasonably matched my other eye. I left the office pretty pleased with my new acquisition.

We drove across town to visit a friend of ours who was pastoring a church in Arlington, a suburb of Jacksonville. I was sitting in his office visiting with him when my newly acquired artificial eye popped out and rested on my cheek. I was slightly perplexed. What should I do? Should I reach up and replace the eye, or should I simply sit there as though everything was just fine. My friend solved the problem for me. "Sam," he said, "would you please put your eye back in your head? It is a little disconcerting to see it staring at me like that." I put it back.

That next Sunday morning I was concluding the service at the church I was pastoring. I had preached what I thought was an incredibly powerful message and had everybody close their eyes and bow their heads for the invitation. After a few moments, I began to close the service with prayer. As I prayed with my head bowed, my right eye exited its socket and dropped quietly onto my Braille Bible, which was opened on the pulpit top in front of me. I did what every other normal person would do. Assuming that everyone had done as I asked, that all had heads bowed and eyes closed, I simply picked up the rogue eye and placed it where it belonged while continuing my closing prayer. As I shook hands with members of the congregation at the exit, one member stated that he appreciated the way I put my eye back without forgetting where I was in my prayer. Obviously, one person was not very obedient.

Three years later, I lost my left eye to the same condition that had caused the loss of the right one. The insurance company finally agreed to allow me to have custom prosthetics made. It was during the process of having them made that I discovered that I had been wearing the stock eye upside down for three years.

The manufacturing of the custom prosthetics, while uncomfortable, was quite interesting. The first step was to make a soft plastic form of my eye socket. This was done by using pliable plastic material with a small plastic stick in the center where the pupil would be located. This material was pushed into my eye socket and manipulated into the internal shape. Warm wax was then injected into the mold with a small needle. It was then manipulated to exactly fill the mold. This took some time and was uncomfortable as the ocularist adjusted the sticks in the center to ensure that the pupils would be even. When this task was completed, the acrylic was poured and the process started over. After the prostheses were baked, Ann was permitted to select the color she liked, and the eyes were painted to her specifications. A few weeks later, we returned to the ocularist's office and picked up some new, pretty blue eyes. Ann loved them!

CHAPTER 14

SOME FINAL THOUGHTS ABOUT MY PARENTS

Things were not always easy in the Thompson household. I remember months on end when Dad could not find work. We ate beans three meals a day. When there was not quite enough to go around, Mom and Dad skipped meals so that we kids could have a little to eat. I remember pay day coming and only one ten pack of hotdogs was purchased for all of us to share. I remember the gas and/or electricity being turned off in the middle of winter because there was not enough money to pay the bills.

I remember something else, though, something that I have carried with me through my entire life of sixty-plus years. I remember that, no matter how little we had, no matter how cold or dark it was in the house, Mom and Dad would turn no person in need away. They were always able to find a little something to eat, even if it was leftover beans and cornbread. There was always an extra blanket, another oil lamp or candle. There was always room for one more.

I especially remember one time that Mom had extended an invitation for a friend of the family to live with us for a while until he got his act together after coming home from Viet Nam. I was quite disturbed when I was told to give up my bed for this guy I did not even know. Mom took me aside and said these gentle words to me. "Sam, it is very important to remember that no matter how little you have, you should never close someone else out. They may have less than you and appreciate what you can offer them. I won't ask you to give up your bed if you really don't want to. We will find someplace else for him to sleep." He slept in my bed, and I slept on the cold floor, willingly.

Mom and Dad showed me what it meant to be hospitable. I was challenged to carry on that tradition when I grew up. Maybe that is why I invited Jane to come by on her way home to Indiana and spend the first night with Ann and me in our new apartment just after we were married. Do you think Ann will buy that excuse? Me neither!

Mom also taught me that there was humor in almost any situation. As I think back on my childhood, there are a number of incidents that would have brought most people to their knees in exasperation. Mom just faced them, stepped back, looked them over, and usually laughed at them. Even when she was having one of her legs amputated in her later years, she looked at the doctor in the operating room and asked him to order her prosthesis with a point on the end so that she could use it to aerate her garden.

Her humor and tenacity have greatly influenced my life. It is in memory of her that I want to end this book with a story from her funeral. Although this was an incredibly sad day for me, it was also the day of one of the funniest things that has ever happened to me, not because the event was so funny, but because I think Mom would have loved what happened.

On the day of Mom's funeral, Ann, Dale, his wife Juanita, and I were sitting on the front row. As we stood to sing the first hymn, one of Mom's favorites, I began to shed a few tears. As I wiped my right eye, my prosthesis dropped out into my handkerchief. I turned to show it to Ann, and then as unobtrusively as possible, put it back into place. I was doing all right until Ann said, "Can you imagine what would have happened if that thing had rolled down the aisle in front of the casket?" We broke up laughing, which prompted Dale to ask what was up. I think the rest of the congregation must have thought we had lost our minds as we stood in the front row of my mom's funeral, doing all we could to control our laughter. It was truly a fitting tribute to a woman who taught me to laugh in the dark.

EPILOGUE

This little book has given you just a small glimpse into my life. There are more stories I could share. Perhaps someday I will write another book. I have made every attempt to ensure that this book is lighthearted, not preachy. In fact, I fear that some of my critics will say that it is not preachy enough. Now, however, I am going to get preachy.

I have wanted to show you some of the humorous things that happened for only one reason. It is my hope that this book will point you to the same source of laughter and happiness I have found. I was an adult before I began to realize that it was okay to laugh at life. I have met many people with disabilities who still have difficulty, but I have met many more who can and do. Our secret? Christ! It was only after we allowed Christ into our lives that we were able to really laugh.

I have made it a practice to listen to people laughing. You can tell a lot about a person by the way he or she laughs. Many are making sounds of laughter, but they do not feel the joy. They are hurting, or they are insecure. They are angry, or they are uncertain. The entertainment industry seeks to make people laugh by providing outlets that feed our sinful needs. A phony joy is trumped up, a reaction to things that are often not really funny. This type of laughter is often filled with cynicism, hate, and anger. On the flip side, the joy that comes from the Lord produces genuine laughter, laughter from the heart, a laughter that says "I am in love with my Lord and with life!"

Which type of laughter do you possess? Are you genuinely laughing, or just going through the motions? If you do not possess the joy of which I speak, this can change. Romans 10:9 says, "If you confess with your mouth, 'Jesus is Lord,' and believe in your heart that God raised Him from the dead, you will be saved" (New International Version). He will turn your mourning into joy. Then, and only then, will you be able to really laugh. No longer will you be going through the motions, laughing in the dark.

FOR ADDITIONAL COPIES OF

LAUGHING IN THE DARK

Contact Sam Thompson at

Clearer Vision Ministries, Inc.
(904) 201-1358

sam@clearervisionministries.org
www.ClearerVisionMinistries.org

(All proceeds from the sale of this book will be used to support the work of Clearer Vision Ministries, Inc.)